D0848330

Saginaw Chippewa Tribal College
2274 Enterprise Drive
Mt. Pleasant, MI 48858

A Gut Feeling

A Gut Feeling

Conquer Your Sweet Tooth by Tuning In to Your Microbiome

Heather Anne Wise

ROWMAN & LITTLEFIELD
Lanham • Boulder • New York • London

Disclaimer: This book is not intended to replace medical diagnosis or treatment, only to aid in tuning in to your own body and to give you the tools to make meaningful changes in your own health.

Published by Rowman & Littlefield
An imprint of The Rowman & Littlefield Publishing Group, Inc.
4501 Forbes Boulevard, Suite 200, Lanham, Maryland 20706
www.rowman.com

Unit A, Whitacre Mews, 26-34 Stannary Street, London SE11 4AB

British Library Cataloguing in Publication Information Available

Library of Congress Cataloging-in-Publication Data Available

ISBN: 978-1-5381-1047-8 (cloth : alk. paper)
ISBN: 978-1-5381-1048-5 (electronic)

∞™ The paper used in this publication meets the minimum requirements of American National Standard for Information Sciences—Permanence of Paper for Printed Library Materials, ANSI/NISO Z39.48-1992.

Printed in the United States of America

For my father,
my inspiration and guidance

Contents

Introduction

In the beginning of my search to uncover the cause of my insistent sugar cravings, I began paying attention to all sorts of strange maladies that I'd previously chosen to ignore. Some symptoms had become so familiar—such as bloat after eating, on-and-off itchy ears and throat, skin issues, and indigestion—that I assumed I would experience them my entire life. Other symptoms were relatively new: chronic fatigue, scattered thoughts, inability to focus, and an insatiable appetite.

I started following possible health clues and researching how these issues as well as symptoms of low blood sugar despite my constant snacking might be connected. In making changes one piece at a time, I started to uncover the intricate causes of my own myriad of ever-increasing, interwoven digestive health problems. Many of the studies I found were buried in academic journals and required a large amount of time to digest—pun intended. At times, I found it necessary to look up medical terms in order to decipher the applicability of these studies to my own life. Study after study was pointing in the same direction: All my symptoms could be connected back to a deficiency of beneficial microbes in the gut and an overgrowth of pathogenic flora.

Researching this further through a medical anthropological lens, I discovered that the average American adult has roughly 1,200 different species of bacteria residing in their gut, while the average Amerindian living in the Amazon of Venezuela has closer to 1,600 species.[1] This gap might just be the key to addressing the epidemic of chronic conditions we face in the United States—compared to the diminutive amount of chronic illness found in less developed countries. In fact, some of the most common foods in the Western diet have been scientifically proven to wreak havoc on our delicate microbial ecosystem and further reduce the number of beneficial microbes residing

1

there, which can trigger a host of other problems—such as a surge in patho-genic fungi.

In an attempt to reflect on my own sugar habits and stress—which were beginning to feel beyond my control—I began to seek comfort in mindful-ness through meditation and yoga. By turning to these practices, rather than to sweets, I found myself beginning to understand the mechanisms in my mind behind my compulsion to eat sweets. I also found myself less self-critical after overdosing on cookies or other tempting, sugar-stuffed snacks. I started to gain more clarity and focus as I recommitted myself, again and again, to cutting back on sugary foods, taking care of my microbiome, and connecting with my body through yoga and mindfulness to regain my whole health. As I gained an awareness of the many species of beneficial flora that live within me and how to foster their growth, and turned away from sugar and other foods fostering the growth of pathogenic flora, I was able to remap my gut ecology, shed weight, and feel a decade younger.

Over time, people took notice of a change in my appearance and energy. They wanted to know what I'd done! The ring of belly fat I'd carried around my waist since childhood seemed to evaporate without any extra exercise or effort, and my face regained its rosy complexion. My foggy thinking disap-peared, my anxiety dwindled, and I stopped getting regular infections. I felt more lively and energetic than ever. I was sleeping better at night and living a more colorful existence during the day. I even found a deeper sense of inner peace and trust in my everyday choices.

Best of all, my sugar cravings were gone, and I felt confident in my food choices. For the first time in my life, I could trust my body's signals. I had a renewed faith in my natural ability to gauge what I needed to eat and to main-tain my new state of health. Now, years after clearing up my health conditions, starting my own health coaching practice, and helping others experience the same benefits to their health and energy as I did years ago, I've condensed all I learned into the following chapters of this book. I hope that my story and the stories of others, backed up with the latest research, can help you reclaim a connection to your body's inner cues so that you can come to trust your own judgment about your body and your health.

NOW IS YOUR TIME

It's time to stop beating yourself up after stuffing your face with sweets or for other bad habits, and to start devoting your full attention to the life you *want* to live rather than the one you don't. Imagine the feeling of freedom when you've accomplished this, and how it will transform your self-image and self-confidence throughout all areas of your life. In what areas of your life do you wish you had the courage and fortitude to do something differently? Taking this first step toward cutting back on sweets will create a ripple effect in all other areas of your life. Now is the time to take charge of your health and live boldly.

The research and stories I present in this book are proof that we *do* have the ability to listen to our bodies and take the necessary steps to change the course of our health and lives. However, we can't just change our diet: We need to change our mind-set, too. It's time to end self-criticisms of your body and bad habits and begin to practice gratitude for your unique body, heart, and mind. During my personal journey with sugar addiction, I discovered that focusing on the outcomes that I wanted to happen was a much more powerful approach than going back over my failures and setbacks. Self-kindness and self-compassion have been integral to healing my own microbiome and addiction to sugar.

My personal journey through sugar addiction and a disrupted microbiome taught me the most invaluable life lesson: By cultivating an awareness of the cues our body is giving us about food cravings and stress, we can develop trust in ourselves—and ultimately become the biggest advocate for our health. That's why I'm not just going to give you a diet plan and tell you that as long as you follow this regimen you will be free of your sugar highs and lows forever. Instead, I will share my research on how to heal the gut and get rid of uncontrollable sweet cravings by adding in a class of foods that have been ignored and scorned for far too long, while giving you tools to manage your stress-induced sweet tooth. I will also share my story of how I healed my gut and navigated through all the obstacles that arose in the process of overcoming my own sugar habits. I'll share the research behind the approach I take with my health coaching clients and provide exercises to support you in setting goals and addressing negative mind-snares that get in the way. Ultimately, though, I leave it up to you to decide for yourself what the best course of action is for your body.

As you read this book, I invite you to reimagine the life you're living and open yourself up to a world of possibilities. You will discover a new way of satisfying your body and your sweet tooth that will allow you to permanently break the cycle of overeating sugary foods. By the end of this book, you will have a newfound understanding of your body, your cravings, and your sweet tooth and will be able to address your eating habits with self-compassion rather than self-criticism. This, in turn, will empower you with the skills to tap into the inner workings of your body and listen to all the signals it is giving you.

Your body is a web of interchanging parts, constantly extracting as many nutrients from your food as it can and using them in thousands of ways to support your body's natural healing processes. It's time to finally begin healing your relationship with food and your body. As you begin to feel differently in your skin, through my diet recommendations and mindfulness exercises, you will start to envision your body as the magnificent system that it is and treat it accordingly. Most importantly, in rebalancing your microbiome you have the opportunity to restore your optimal health and sustainably care for your unique physical body for years to come.

• 1 •

Wake-Up Call

I remember that day vividly. Staring at my reflection in the mirror, I submitted to my inner truth, finally listening to the little voice inside of me telling me that something was wrong—I could no longer deny it. Despite having dealt with indigestion, infections, anxiety, and sugar cravings for years, my symptoms had escalated to a whole new level. My skin had been pasty for so many months I'd cultivated a habit of relying on blush and lipstick every morning to appear rosy and healthy. Although sleeping twelve- to thirteen-hour nights had become the new norm, I never felt rested. My head was constantly foggy and my attention scattered. With the occasional dizzy spells and weak immune system—judging from the biweekly stomach bugs, sore throats, and yeast infections—I started to fear the worst. Looking at my belly, I saw the all-too-familiar disproportionate amount of tummy fat, despite staying very active through running and yoga and by walking most places. What's more, I felt bloated after every meal, and—what should have been my first clue—*my sugar cravings were stronger than ever.*

That was just the beginning. I'd also started to notice strange maladies that didn't make sense. My hands and feet were always freezing, my tongue had developed a permanent, whitish coating, and the tightness in my chest had become so commonplace that I couldn't remember what it felt like *not* to be anxious all the time. In fact, finding short-term relief through exercise only made me realize how pervasive my anxiety was in every nook and cranny of my life. It frustrated me that I had all these ailments in the first place, when I devoted so much energy to my health.

How had it come to this?

When I went to my primary care physician with my list of ailments, I got a shrug. My doctor had no experience dealing with my list of seemingly unrelated symptoms. I went from doctor to doctor, but it was always the same. Each time, I'd leave with only a handwritten note for an over-the-counter treatment from a local pharmacy for my yeast infection and a referral to a psychologist for my anxiety. I felt frustrated and at a loss for what to do about my ever-increasing laundry list of problems. *If there is really nothing to be done now, how am I to avoid more serious health issues down the road?* This was not the type of preventative care I was seeking.

I was much too young—only twenty-two—to be having all these problems. My health symptoms prevented me from doing many activities women this age are drawn to. I couldn't stay out drinking with friends because I'd get so bloated my stomach appeared three months prenatal. I couldn't really stay out late at all, for that matter, because I was constantly fatigued. I thought the stress of finals and my senior year of college might be the cause, but as the end of the school year came and went, my health did not improve. I quickly realized that I needed to take matters into my own hands if I wanted to get better. I knew sweets were bad for me in general, but my out-of-control sweet cravings waking me in the middle of the night and trailing me throughout the day felt like a freight train I couldn't stop.

I knew what was going wrong was tied to my digestive system, yet I believed I was a healthy eater. I'd felt liberated when I moved into an off-campus apartment earlier in the year. For the first time in my life, I was 100 percent in charge of the food I ate. The possibilities to cook and prepare foods that made me feel nourished and energized seemed endless. After a lifetime of school cafeteria food and living among three brothers who devoured almost everything brought home from the grocery store in a matter of hours—leaving me scrounging between meals to find any food at all—I faithfully made a habit of stocking and cooking delicious foods in the kitchen I now called my own. I relished mundane tasks like doing my own shopping, organizing my pantry, and preparing meals on my own time and to my own preference. Even having the ability to set the mood for my meals in my sparse kitchen with dim lighting and soft music felt like an honor.

Despite all this, nearing the end of my senior year of college, standing in my bathroom, my feet cold and bare on the tile floor, I stared at my reflection in the mirror in confusion. My pallid complexion stared back at me, devoid of life and color.

Do something, it seemed to whisper. I let out a sigh of frustration.

I had been doing everything I could to lead a healthy lifestyle and prevent illness. I'd kept a well-balanced diet, and I didn't smoke, eat fast food, or drink soda. How could there be anything wrong with my health? My meals regularly consisted of foods such as granola, sautéed kale, vegetable or bean soup, spelt pasta, eggs, smoked salmon, boiled buckwheat groats, butter, avocados, and locally baked bread, often with a slice of aged cheddar on top. My sweet fixes weren't even as bad as they were for some of my friends. My cravings were frequent, but I fed them mostly with dark chocolate from the local discount natural food store, organic cookies, graham crackers, cereals, fruit, bran muffins, and sweetened yogurts. *These are "healthy" sweets, right?* I thought so, yet I found myself questioning the validity of this statement.

The truth was, wheat and sugar were what I desired most and the only foods that could satisfy my sweet cravings at the time. I would look forward to long hours spent studying at a local café as an excuse to get what I considered a well-deserved scone or cupcake to go with my café latte. As long as most of my sugar fixes were made from whole grain and/or organic flour, I did not consider them unhealthy. I'd also developed a habit of having a glass of red wine most nights to wind down, since I was now finally old enough to purchase alcohol, which felt like a privilege after years of surreptitious drinking as an undergrad. *Besides, I reasoned, wine is a good source of antioxidants.* My diet seemed reasonable, especially given my active lifestyle, so I hadn't put much thought into how it related to my ongoing symptoms. After all, I'd been living with most of these symptoms since high school and had learned how to tune them out most of the time. *So what if I eat cookies every day, often have a drink to wind down, and crave sugar all the time,* I'd tell myself. *Overall, I'm eating very healthy, so it cancels out all the sugar.*

Yet, backtracking in my mind, I started to realize how my attempts at balancing healthy foods and sweet foods were not working. I couldn't deny that I felt a little out of control when it came to the sweet foods and processed, refined grains in my diet.

Despite my newfound freedom and freshly printed degree in hand, I felt distracted and cornered by all my chronic health issues lurking in the background. I called my mother, expecting her to know what was wrong with me—she was a holistic medical doctor, after all. Her response was somewhat vague, but it gave me a hint that I could run with. She said, "It could have something to do with an overgrowth of *Candida* in your gut, honey." But she couldn't explain what *Candida* was very clearly and didn't seem to be well versed in the delicate internal environment of the microbiome, an uncommon term in the medical world at the time. Let alone how the microbiome affected blood sugar or sugar cravings. I was on my own.

I had lived under the illusion that I was perfectly healthy for as long as I could remember, when all this time I'd been hiding from a part of myself I didn't want to face. I'd developed a reputation for my health expertise among my college friends and prided myself on my research and nutrition knowledge, gladly sharing it with anyone who wanted to listen, but I was completely stumped when it came to my own symptoms. It was impossible to think that

I could be so blind to such a chronic health problem for so long. Yet looking myself square in the eye for the first time, a slightly overweight, exhausted, sugar-addicted, vulnerable side of me stared back.

Swallowing my pride, I made a new lifelong commitment to myself that day—*to start listening to my own inner voice that urged me to eat and live in a whole new way, as if my life depended on it.* That day I finally began listening to the *inner* gut feelings I'd had my whole life around eating, instead of the looming, often overpowering *external* social cues that had been influencing and shaping my life and diet for decades.

I immediately began to follow up on my symptoms with scientific and public health research, consultation with GI tract experts and holistic doctors, and documented my findings. Like a detective in my own mystery novel, I began to write down what was I eating and what symptoms came as a result. These clues led to more clues, one after the next, until they all started to fit together.

My first clue that something was off with both my blood sugar and my digestive system lay in how quickly I found myself hungry—and not just hungry, but *starving.* Within only a couple of hours after eating a substantial meal, I would feel a signal of high alert run through my body, telling me it was time to eat again. I'd get hunger pangs so strong it felt like my stomach was tying itself into knots trying to squeeze every last morsel of nutrition out. I'd grab a quick snack to quench the hunger, only to go through the same cycle a few hours later.

I started to closely observe exactly what I was eating and took notes on how each food affected my sugar cravings and hunger pangs afterward. I referred to the "glycemic index," which measures how a carbohydrate-containing food raises blood glucose levels.[1] The lower the score, the better that food is in stabilizing blood sugar. Broccoli scores a low 10 on the glycemic scale, while white table sugar typically scores from 60 to 75. I soon realized that my diet contained a large amount of foods high or medium on the glycemic scale, such as bread, cereal, and other refined grains.

I knew from my nutrition studies in college that I was definitely eating more than I needed throughout the day, so why was I always so hungry? After monitoring my intake for a few weeks, I discovered that even a small amount of a "healthy" high-glycemic food, such as a slice of artisanal white bread, when eaten on an empty stomach, was sending my blood sugar on a roller-coaster ride leading to the all too familiar feeling of bloat, fatigue, and sugar cravings. What goes up must come down! The more closely I observed the cause and effect relationship with sweets and refined grains, the more undeniable my imbalanced blood sugar became. This was hard to accept, given my devotion to an organic, whole grain, whole food diet. What had gone wrong?

The possibility that I could have slightly imbalanced blood sugar wasn't shocking. My father had been diagnosed as pre-diabetic in his early forties, and my grandma had passed away from complications related to diabetes when I was four years old. Metabolic disorders, such as inflammation, ran rampant in my immediate and extended family. But how could I be having blood sugar issues without being diabetic?

These days, people with "perfect" blood sugar levels are like four-leaf clovers in a jungle of crabgrass. In fact, having "perfect" blood sugar levels is becoming rarer and rarer. Currently, 50 percent of the people in the United States struggle with a diagnosed blood sugar imbalance in the form of pre-diabetes, hyperglycemia, and type 1 or type 2 diabetes—characterized by a fasting blood sugar level of 100 mg/dL or higher.[2] An even larger portion of the population has undiagnosed pre-diabetes, or mildly unstable blood sugar, which puts them at a high risk for developing diabetes. The Centers for Disease Control and Prevention (CDC) says that at least 86 million Americans—almost one in three—have pre-diabetes, which is marked by blood sugar levels that are higher than normal, but not high enough to qualify as diabetic.[3] By these estimates, well over half the entire population has some form of blood sugar disequilibrium, and 90 percent of them don't even know it.[4]

Slowly, I started to remove high-glycemic foods such as refined grains like wheat and sweets from my diet. I said goodbye to mainstream pasta, bread, muffins, cereal, candy, ice cream, and even 100 percent fruit juice and replaced these sweets with things like spelt and almond flour pumpkin muffins, brown rice, millet porridge, chickpea flour pancakes, green smoothies sweetened with ripe banana, avocado chocolate pudding, and coconut cream sweetened with raw honey and topped with blueberries.

The results were immediate. I start noticing many of my symptoms clearing up within days. I was no longer bloated after every meal and starving a few hours later. My head was clearer, my attention span longer, my yeast infections fewer and farther between. With my ravenous food cravings abating, I found I had so much more energy!

Excited at my progress, I turned my attention to my digestive system. Research in journals and consultations with holistic doctors, including my mother, led me to the discovery that my gut bacteria—or lack of it, in fact—could be an even deeper underlying factor.

What if I told you that everything we thought unchangeable—our metabolism, chronic pain, digestive upset, fatigue, taste buds and food cravings, even our personality traits—were all due to microscopic beings influencing every emotion, physical sensation, and experience coming from within our bodies. Science is discovering that who we think we are largely is due to the composition of microbes within us. The microbiome has been defined as the entire collection of genes found in all the microbes within the human body. The genetic makeup of microbes is as unique as a fingerprint. Our microbial genes outnumber our human genes by 100 to 1. We inherit roughly 20,000 to 25,000 genes from our parents, while we inherit well over 3 million genes from our environment in the form of bacteria and other microbes.[5] If you think there may be a genetic link to a health outcome in your family, remember that 99.9 percent of the genes in your body come not from parental DNA but from exposure to microbes—often the same bacteria your parents are exposed to, thus creating a similar microbiome. And 99 percent of all those microbial genes reside in our gut.[6] We've long known that the microbial makeup of our intestinal microbes can alter gene expression in our gut, including genes involved in immunity, nutrient absorption, energy metabolism, and resiliency of the gut barrier to prevent "leaky gut."[7] Recent findings from the Fred Hutchinson Cancer Research Center and the University of Washington have shown that our dietary metabolism and the resulting microbial makeup of our gut likely even influence gene expression of our parental DNA.[8]

It's our gut—not our brain, our heart, or our human DNA, as many people think—that's actually in charge. The gut acts as a central control panel underlying our central nervous system, unconscious cravings and desires, and other physical processes affecting both our physical and mental health. Unlike a fingerprint, though, this composition of bacteria, fungi, and other microbes in our gut is constantly changing as a result of stress levels, medications, diet, personal relationships, pets, and environmental exposures. In fact, it wouldn't be too far off to say that essentially everything you come into contact with, both physically and emotionally, will impact your health by having either a positive or negative impact on the symbiotic microbes in your gut.

Scientific literature has connected a weakened microbiome—termed *dysbiosis*, or altered microbes—to a weakened immune system, weight gain, systemic inflammation, inflammatory bowel disease, diabetes, metabolic disease, and many more chronic conditions.[9, 10] For years, modern medicine has linked systemic inflammation with chronic illnesses such as cardiovascular disease, type 2 diabetes, obesity, gastrointestinal disorders, and more. Only now are we starting to understand that systemic inflammation often begins with an imbalanced microflora.[11]

Another way to think about the microbiome is as an ecosystem of microbes within and on the human body, or the collection of microbes that live in your human "habitat." The biodiversity within our intestines is similar to any ecosystem—the more diverse the species, the greater its health. When biodiversity of flora and fauna diminishes, opportunistic, invasive species can take over, resulting in an imbalanced microbiome. In the case of our gut flora, as the diversity of various strains of bacteria and fungi is reduced, pathogenic strains of bacteria and fungi such as *Candida* tend to flourish.[12] Unlike the beneficial microbes and other helpful flora in our bodies, overgrowth of *Candida albicans* can lead to blood sugar imbalances, causing the drops in blood sugar that result in sugar cravings.[13] *Candida albicans* is just one of the hundreds of thousands of strains of flora that make up the human body's microbiome. A small amount is harmless, but when gut bacteria biodiversity has been weakened due to use of certain medications and foods, *Candida* overgrowth is common.

Having studied anthropology and environmental studies in college, this analogy made perfect sense to me. In a river ecosystem, the rapid overgrowth of one invasive species of underwater fern can threaten the survival of other underwater plants as it conquers more and more territory. Soon fish and bacteria, also a part of this delicate ecosystem, and reliant on the sunlight that is now blocked by the tentacles of the large fern overgrowth, start to die off. Similarly, an overgrowth of pathogenic fungi in our gut microbiome will negatively affect all the other microbes living in the body and, by extension, our metabolism, immune system, and expression of our genes. Eureka!

Despite the potential harm of various gut-damaging exposures, which we will get into later, the type of gut flora that dominates the space in your gut is strongly influenced by what you eat. One recent study from the journal *Nutrients* stated, "Diet has the most powerful influence on gut microbial communities in healthy human subjects."[14] We need to eat the type of food that our healthy, immune-boosting flora love, not the type that kills the diversity and feeds pathogenic strains of bacteria and fungi. According to Stig Bengmark, MD, PhD, honorary visiting professor in surgery and interventional science at the University College London, "About 75 percent of the food in the Western diet is of limited or no value to the (beneficial) microbiota of the lower gut" due to its limited amounts of minerals, vitamins, fiber, and other nutrients our beneficial flora feast on.[15]

Eating and living in a whole new way is easier said than done, but our microbes also play a huge role in our taste buds and food cravings. Because it is possible to change our microbial disposition through diet and lifestyle, it is also possible to alter many of our taste buds and food cravings. By changing our gut microbe diversity, we can help our bodies crave more whole foods and naturally sweet foods such as organic apples or berries, as opposed to processed, refined sugars, positively altering our body disposition as a result.

MY MOTIVATION TO UNCOVER THE TRUTH

Sugar was my habit and my vice for many years, but it was also my comfort, my self-medication for stress and fatigue—and my self-reward when I accomplished something of which I was proud. *How could I cut out something so deeply embedded in my life?* Deep down I knew it was not going to be easy for me. Cutting out sugar for a period of time would help, but I realized the road would be long to completely restore my microbial health.

In my detective mind, I saw my sweet cravings as a major clue to my health problems. I wanted to understand this compulsion from a scientific and psychological perspective. When my sweet cravings hit, the thought of having something sweet could be so overpowering I couldn't focus on anything until I had that snack food in my hand. A little sleuthing revealed that a pleasurable memory, no matter what it is, leaves a permanent imprint in the prefrontal cortex region of the brain. In the beginning stages, this is how many addictive habits are formed, long before there are any longer-term chemical alterations in the brain or in the makeup of microbes in the gut. Whether it's a healthy habit like a runner's high, or an unhealthy one for sugary sweets, memory is a powerful factor that causes us to replay that pleasurable experience in our minds and yearn to re-create it. It's hard to attempt to inhibit the replay of that pleasurable memory, or even recognize that our brain is hitting replay without our permission, causing us to reach for that experience as if on autopilot.

Ironically, I discovered it's also the job of the prefrontal cortex to inhibit unhealthy impulses that we know have consequences. My first experiment from my research on how the brain works was to motivate my prefrontal cortex to stay away from sweets by making a list of all the negative outcomes I wanted to prevent—weight gain, fatigue, feeling bloated, and all the symptoms associated with an overgrowth of fungi (oversleeping, scattered and unfocused thinking, yeast infections, etc.). I figured I just needed to trick my prefrontal cortex into focusing on the ill effects in order to prevent myself from giving into the impulse to buy sweets. A negative plus a positive cancel each other out, right? Wrong. Unfortunately, focusing on the negative side effects of eating sugar turned out to be the opposite of motivating. This focus ended up backfiring, leading me to feel more depressed as a result of these self-criticisms, which then caused me to reach for sugar to lift my mood! By focusing on my health problems, I was actually re-creating those negative memories in my mind, continuing to feel trapped by them, and unconsciously repeating the same behaviors that caused them in the first place. Unsurprisingly, my brain preferred to re-create a positive thought, such as eating a sweet treat, much more than a laundry list of health problems.

I changed direction and tried another technique—focusing on what I wanted to happen. This technique replaced the positive memory of eating sweets with an even more positive image of what it would be like once I stopped eating sweets for a few months. I imagined losing weight, feeling great in my body and skin, gaining confidence, and having everything turn up in my life. It turns out that one positive can only be replaced by another positive. It was like a light went on in my brain, and I felt a good, wholesome, motivating boost of energy. *This is what true motivation feels like*, I thought to myself.

I started to make long lists of how my life would change once I stopped eating sugar and refined foods. This list included things such as feeling delicious and confident in my body, feeling my clothes cling to my shoulders and hips rather than my stomach, feeling centered and focused rather than scattered and foggy, being a role model to those I care about so they can adopt healthy behaviors too, having the energy to pursue my highest aspirations, and on and on. Eventually I aligned my goal to cut sugar out of my diet with all the things I valued and desired the most in my life, such as my health, my relationships, my confidence, and being more loving and accepting of my body.

WRITING INTENTIONS

Take a moment now and write down a list of all your intentions for freeing yourself from the tight grip of unhealthy food or sweet cravings. Why do you want to be free of these cravings? Write how you see your life changing once you are. How will this transform your health, your daily life, and your relationships in a positive way? Don't hold back! The sky is the limit here.

TAKEAWAYS

- All too often the foods we crave the most, and are the most addicted to, may be the same ones wreaking havoc in our body.
- Finding out what we care about the most and aligning our goal to cut out unhealthy foods with those values is the most powerful way to change habits.

Eat to fuel myself.
Not fall out of control
Enjoy meals + be full
Not be scared for my bf to touch me
Positive relationship with food

Mirrors
Wearing sports bras without hating my arm fat

• *2* •

Sweet Intentions

As we must account for every idle word, so must we account for
every idle silence.

—Benjamin Franklin

*M*y first attempts to listen to my gut and tune back in to my body left me
feeling lost and confused about my own body's needs. I was eating plenty
of food, but it seemed as if my body was starving and craving sugar almost
constantly. Yet my body's physical cues weren't the only thing that had my
head spinning. A small-town girl from the East Coast, I had moved across
the country after college and was desperate to make friends in a new world
far from home. This desire all too often led me to focus too much attenion
on helping others rather than taking a look at my own life and making the
changes to become who I wanted to be. If we are sacrificing our own inner
needs to care for someone else, we can burn out very quickly. Anyone who
has kids understands how important it is to take time to recharge and reconnect with one's own self-care each day. I learned this lesson the hard way even
before I had my daughter. On a deep level I didn't trust I could find my own
source of happiness within me, and so I looked outside myself by turning to
sugar, food, guys, family, good causes, friends, travel, work . . . but this was
where it went wrong.

Somewhere along the way, while trying to please everyone around me,
I had stopped taking proper care of my own body—what should have always
been my first priority—and started to lose my connection with my own inner
voice—the place inside me that always knew what I needed in the moment.
Some may think of this place as our heart or soul. If we take a look biologi-
cally, this physical and emotional resilience might largely stem from our gut,
where our gut microbes are making the chemicals and neurotransmitters we

require to feel grounded, strong, and content even amid stress or trauma. This in turn sends messages of calm and safety from our enteric nervous system, or second brain located in the gut, through the vagus nerve to our brain and the rest of our body.

This was the beginning, for me, of learning how to master the replenishment of my own internal microbial reserves. By putting my health above all else and communicating these needs with those around me, I started to learn how to give myself the attention I was so desperate to receive from others. Ironically, learning how to understand my own body's cues taught me how to better provide quality attention and care not only to myself, but also to those I loved. By acknowledging my gut's discord, a part of me I had denied for so many years, I was finally acknowledging my own gut brain and what it had been trying to tell me all my life—how to truly listen to my body. I began to tune in to my body on a daily basis through introspective journaling, mindful eating, meditation, and yoga, all the while weeding out the foods and activities that were making me feel bloated, lethargic, disconnected, and sick.

Sugar was still making me feel sick, yet I fought with myself over and over. I knew that I shouldn't be eating sugary foods, but all too often my sugar cravings, fueled by my sugar-loving microbiome, spoke louder than the truth lying underneath. My mind would often come up with some excuse to give in: *It's okay to have a cookie now, you can just start the sugar detox and balance your gut tomorrow, after the party.* Or other times: *Just have one cocktail or else people will wonder why you're not drinking*—arguments like this would run on and on in my head. My self-persuasion was very convincing. I'd try for a week and then give in to a huge piece of chocolate cake my boyfriend would bring home for me as a seemingly *nice* gesture. It's amazing how quickly my internal commitment would crumble, compromising my own integrity and trust in myself, and forcing me to start the process all over again. I could not even bring myself to set a clear boundary and ask him to stop bringing me cake! The voice of sugar-fueled persuasion was filling my head and muffling the healthy microbes (which live off prebiotic foods) screaming in starvation underneath.

Developing a new set of flora that will crave flora-friendly foods is possible. There is a learning curve, but soon it will become difficult to turn away from these new healthy habits. It all starts in your microbiome. As hard as it is to imagine, there's an entire world of flora and fauna living inside you with its own needs and desires—and what your internal ecosystem wants, you'll want too. You are both inseparable. Evolutionarily, bacteria and other microbes thrive and grow best by influencing us to choose foods that contain the nutrients they need to survive.[1] Unfortunately, this holds true for both beneficial flora and pathogenic strains. How do they accomplish this feat?

There is a whole field of study exploring how bacteria and fungi affect the neural signals along the vagus nerve, which travels from our large intestine, wrapping around our stomach along the way, up to our brain. Some microbes can release toxins that make us feel bad when we are not eating what they want us to. On the flip side, when we eat their favorite foods, they reward us with chemicals that make us feel good—all in the interest of their own survival.[2] One thing our microbiota has the biggest control over is our food cravings. There is a specific strain of bacteria or fungi that favors every single food we put in our bodies.[3] Some love tea, some love asparagus, some spinach or onions, and some—like *Candida albicans*—love sugar. What you eat and how you live has a huge effect on the specific strains of microorganisms inhabiting your intestines. This community within affects your moods, your desires, your cravings, and your actions.

Within the intestinal enteric nervous system, neurons are connected in networks, just like in our brain. When those networks fire we perceive, feel, think, reason, and act. As we feel a certain way, those networks get worn in— like steps in a forest slowly wear into a path. The neurons that fire together wire together and eventually become habit—a well-worn trail in our mind and body. If you take steps toward changing that world of bacteria and other microbes inside you, this in turn will alter neural networks within your enteric nervous system, sending new messages to your brain so that you crave different things. How is this possible? It is hypothesized that the microbes within our gastrointestinal tract behave like an organ, supplying our enteric nervous system with neurons.[4] In this light, our nervous system is driving our composition of microbial flora while our microbes are communicating with our nervous system to dictate what the microbial population needs for its own survival. It's a two-way street! For example, as we shift our mind-set and change our brain chemistry through mindfulness practices, these benefits extend to our gut. If we can then tune in to the healthy microbes and listen to what they are telling us, we can rebuild our microflora and restore our physical and mental health. The first step is figuring out whether the signals and cravings coming from your gut are coming from the healthy or the pathogenic flora residing there. But once you understand what the unhealthy strains are telling you to eat, as we will go over in this book, that's not too difficult.

No matter what your distracting unhealthy cravings are telling you, just remember that's their job, to keep you eating and living in the exact same way you've been eating, so your current microbial mix will remain unchanged. When we change our diet, we change our microbiome, which in turn changes our genes and our biology and results in new food cravings, improved metabolism, and more efficient nutrient absorption. And it all happens much quicker than you would think.

DEVELOPING CONSCIOUS INTENTION

Rather than counting calories or giving exact instruction on what to eat at each meal, my approach to healing an imbalance in the gut with my health coaching clients starts with two initial phases: (1) understanding the role of gut flora, and (2) developing conscious intention in diet and lifestyle habits. Let's take a deeper look at the intentions behind our everyday choices.

Our feelings and thoughts lead to the personal choices we make. When we acknowledge and understand how we are feeling or why we are thinking a certain way, we can understand what is motivating our actions. Conscious or unconscious, I would argue that everything—and I mean *everything*—we do, we do with motivation or intention. Whether we are aware of our intentions or not, they are the true driving force behind our actions. If my only motivation when I choose my lunch options during a busy day is to get something quick and cheap, whether or not I acknowledge this is my priority, this focus will be the main intention behind my food choices, and I will most likely end up with something that is low quality and cheap. However, if I set a new intention to fill my body with nutrients to energize me for the rest of the day and to feel satisfied without going over budget, then I will probably end up choosing a delicious, affordable, whole foods–based meal.

It's easy to accomplish our intentions when we set out with a single objective and don't see any obstacles. *Perfect, my schedule is free tonight—I'm going to go to yoga today after work and get to bed early!* The very act of performing an activity of self-care that aligns with our values bolsters our sense of integrity and improves our self-esteem or self-worth, the part of ourselves that knows deep down we are going to be okay despite all the difficulties in our lives. Ben Franklin, Buddha, and Aristotle believed that one's integrity is the truest and most reliable source of happiness and fulfillment in one's life. In Benjamin Franklin's words, this internal faith and trust in our own abilities is what breeds integrity. The more internal trust we build, the more we improve our self-worth and the more confident we are to go out into the world and get what we want. It's the ideal symbiotic dynamic, which we can create within ourselves for happiness and success. Our sense of self-worth is a necessary grounding force that moves us in the direction of our greatest vision for our lives.

What exactly builds trust in oneself? Telling yourself you are going to take better care of yourself and then taking the necessary steps to do so is one of the easiest, most surefire ways you can build trust and self-worth. If you value taking care of your body and cultivating a sense of well-being, then just the act of purchasing this book is a step that aligns with your values and thereby builds your integrity. All the time and energy you put into learning how to better care for yourself—by subsequently reading this book after purchasing it—exponentially moves you in the direction of success. Reading, dare I say, any book on the topic of gut health or wellness is therefore going to build your confidence and create positive thoughts and mind-sets around healing your gut and improving your health. In the early days of my first sugar detox, as I continued the process of recommitting again and again to avoiding sugar, I began strengthening my faith in myself. I refused to give up on my body. One day I found myself taking just one bite of cake at a party and throwing the rest away, as I promised myself I would. I was so proud of myself I felt like jumping for joy.

Of course, it gets more complicated when we have multiple intentions or motivations that conflict with one another. *I want to go to the gym because I know it's good for my health, but I also value spending time with my family when I get home from work.* In this case, we may set the intention to go to the gym, but it conflicts with our value of spending quality time with our kids, and the stronger value will win out. When you find that some of your goals conflict with strong values you have, it's time to reexamine what is really most important to you and alter your goals slightly. In other words, whatever you are most passionate about doing is what you need to pursue to build your sense of integrity and take steps toward fulfillment in life.

This concept may sound simple, but if someone were to walk up to you right now and ask what your top ten values were, in order, you might fumble a bit. It is sometimes tough to identify and prioritize your values. This could be one of the most important exercises you ever learn how to do, and it is very easy.

I want you to take a moment right now to write down five values that you want to pursue and strengthen in your life—things that you want to move toward, that empower you, that make you feel fulfilled (e.g., good habits, supportive relationships, healthy behaviors, etc.). Next, write down five values that you want to move away from or eliminate from your life. These are things that drain you, that make you regret your actions (e.g., bad habits, negative relationships, and unhealthy behaviors, etc.).

For the five positive values, I want you to write down five actual steps you are taking to support those behaviors. For example, if your positive value was, *Having a good relationship with my family*, then you could write down how you make a point to spend evenings and weekends with your family. The idea is to give a concrete example of your value.

Lastly, I want you to write down five actual steps that you are taking to move away from your five negative values. These steps should be clear examples of how you are attempting to stop, remove, or change your negative

Table 2.1. Values and Actions Chart

Personal values, habits, and relationships I want to move away from.	Personal values, habits, and relationships I want to move *toward* in my life.
Concrete examples and steps I have taken to move away from these negative values, habits, and relationships.	Concrete examples and steps I have taken to move toward these positive values, habits, and relationships.

values, habits, and relationships. For example, if a negative habit that you want to move away from is, *I want to stop blaming others and take responsibility for my own actions*, you might recall a time you said to your partner, "I'm sorry I walked away from you; I'm committed to talking things through."

For these last two steps, be careful to be honest with yourself. Look carefully at each action to see if it really lines up with your values. Notice if you cannot find a clear action that supports your inner value. This is good information and an opportunity for change.

Think about the Values and Actions Chart as a snapshot of your personal values at this moment (see Table 2.1). These are things that have likely been on your mind, taking up mental space and motivating a good amount of your behavior. They are the foundation of your present intentions. Carl Jung once said, "Until you make the unconscious conscious, it will direct your life, and you will call it fate." Think about this chart as a way to start making your intentions more of a conscious choice. Take one or more of these values and make a real goal for yourself, then put it in your calendar. If it's a priority, it needs a regular space in your busy schedule. Here's an example:

Table 2.2. My Values and Health Goals

My Values	Spending quality time with family, being physically fit and strong, having freedom with choices, helping those in need, being a good mother
My Health Goals	Old Goal: ~~Go to the gym every day after work for forty minutes for one month to stay active and strong.~~ New Goal: Take my daughter to the park every day after work (twenty-minute brisk walk each way) for one month to stay active and strong.

As you can see in my chart, I've changed my earlier stated goal of going to the gym every day after work to walking my daughter in the stroller to the park every day. My new goal gets me forty minutes of brisk walking every day, plus it hits four of my values in one—being physically fit and strong, being a good mother, helping those in need (kids do *need* to play outside), and spending quality time with family. Maybe I could even try to hit another value while I'm accomplishing my goal, such as trying out different parks, thus hitting my value of having freedom in my choices and not feeling confined to visiting just one park every day. Remember, the more values you can hit with a single health or wellness goal, the more motivation you will have to accomplish what you've set out to do!

FEAR, OUR BEST AND WORST FRIEND

We all know a few things we could be doing differently to live a happier, healthier life. So what gets in the way? Fear wields its power, like a whisper in our ear, telling us we can't achieve what we set out to do because we're not rich enough, not loved enough, not smart enough, not talented enough, not *something* enough. We may not even be aware of our most deeply instilled fears, and yet they wield more power over our daily choices than we can imagine. If we are feeling overly tired and lackluster in the first place, often due to a weakened microbiome, then it can be easy to give in to these voices of self-doubt. Let's go through some of the excuses we often give ourselves for not eating well when we are physically or mentally drained: too busy, too tired, too poor, too depressed, can't bake, can't cook. These are all just excuses that we convince ourselves are true. The reality is, you create your life; no one else does. When you're taking steps toward healing your microbiome, you are simultaneously making the decision to become more mindful of your body and your actions, and there simply isn't space for these exhausted, age-old excuses.

Fear, which for me comes in the form of stomach pain, indigestion, anxiety, and fatigue, has been present throughout my journey trying to heal my gut and get my life on track. Its coaxing voice sounds something like this: *Now, now, life is hard, you deserve a reward for all that you put up with. Just kick your feet up and enjoy a nice sweet, you'll feel so much better.* Sound familiar? Of course, I never *did* feel better by eating stimulating sweets when I was already feeling anxious or had a stomachache! I often just felt guilty, bloated, and weaker and more tired from the blood sugar drop I endured after giving in to sugar's temptation once again.

Fear is an enabler for many of our unhealthy habits. For me, it was a voice inside my mind that was flat-out terrified of straying from the well-worn paths of familiarity, and its best friend—sugar—just kept sweet-talking me for years, promising I would feel better, that all my troubles and fatigue would melt away, albeit temporarily, in the bite of a cookie. The logic behind thinking of sugar as "therapeutic" is indeed a trick, and quite a dangerous thought, because in fact it is the opposite of what we often really need in the moment. If we are tired after a long day, we need to rest, not consume a stimulant like sugar! It will only further our exhaustion due to the eventual blood sugar drop, disruption to our microbiome, and strain on our liver. If I truly wanted to do something caring and replenishing for my body, I could choose from so many other options, such as an Epsom salt bath with my favorite music in the background, or making herbal tea sweetened with natural microbe-friendly sweeteners like 100 percent monk fruit or stevia. Once I got to a place internally where I recognized the trick sugar had been playing on me all those years, I could consciously choose not to listen to this voice and instead do something that both quelled my anxiety and soothed my stomach, restoring my healthy microbial balance once again.

There is a biological reason we often turn to food for comfort. Ghrelin, a chemical released by your body to send a signal that you have had enough to eat, is also released when you feel safe. In primitive times, having a full stomach meant that you could take a rest from the hard work of hunting or gathering food. It also meant that your tribe and family were going to be okay for a little while. The next time you hear this familiar pull to eat for comfort, instead do something empowering that also helps you feel safe and comforted. Share your feelings with a close friend, or make yourself a cup of herbal tea and write down all that's going through your mind. Take a walk in nature, meditate, take a hot bath, or just relax. Choose an activity that brings a renewed self-awareness about what's driving you to yet again reach for a chocolate bar or other sugary food in the first place. Here's a response to give those persuasive voices in your head: *No thank you, fear, I know you are just trying to keep me safe, but I'm ready to take a leap of faith and change the course of my life, so I've got it from here.* By turning away from negative self-talk that feeds self-doubts and attachment to sugar, you are actually teaching yourself one of the most valuable skills you'll ever learn—how to tune in to your inner microbes and respond with choices that will set the course of your health and life in the direction you want. Let's not forget, we have the capacity to change our genes with the food we eat—that's a pretty powerful thing! Every time your unhealthy gut flora win the debate on what to eat or put in your body, you are in trouble. Every time your beneficial flora win out, however, you are resetting the control panel of your body in the direction of well-being in every sense of the word—health, positive mood, confidence, and a boost to your integrity.

CHERISH YOUR THIN SKIN

We form many of our strongest unconscious beliefs about ourselves and the world around us before we can even talk. During the first three years of life, a child's brain triples in weight and establishes over 1,000 trillion nerve connections, including millions more in the gut and enteric nervous system. As babies, our reptilian brain's emotional response to situations forms unconscious understandings that we carry with us into adulthood. Our most powerful memories and beliefs are cemented into the most primitive part of our brain—the brain stem—in the first twenty-five years of our life, before our cerebral cortex, which is responsible for rational thought, is fully developed.

In a busy household with two working parents and four kids close in age, directly or indirectly I formed the unconscious belief, probably starting around age three, that my feelings and emotions were not of value and were in fact a burden to those around me. Not having learned the words to put to my own emotions, coupled with negative feedback after sharing my emotions, made communicating those emotions to others increasingly frustrating and aggravating—to the point that I became an angry child and threw fits often. This perceived sense of feeling like a burden only got stronger as I grew older, given that my parents were overwhelmed, often stuck in survival mode just trying to pay the bills and raise four kids in the midst of running their own small business. The fact that my emotions were often ignored unless I screamed or yelled to get my parents' attention—which granted me the coveted undivided attention just for a moment, even if I was punished—only reinforced my belief as a child that my feelings were not valued. As I entered adulthood, in relationship after relationship I failed to recognize how sharing my vulnerabilities and feelings with those closest to me actually strengthened the feeling of connection between us, which in turn helped my partner value me more. This was opposite of what I had experienced growing up. By not sharing my vulnerabilities, even into my adult years, I was actually creating more isolation and distance between myself and those I cared for, which reinforced my belief that my feelings were not important. All without realizing that this limiting belief was sabotaging my relationships along with my health! The answer for me was to practice authentic self-love regularly, challenging the core belief that addressing my true feelings was not worth my time or energy. By consciously taking time to prepare homemade meals, experimenting with different fermented foods and green smoothie recipes, and doing mindful activities like yoga and meditation, I began to create rituals that slowly built my self-worth on a daily basis. My internal commitment to my gut health requires me to continuously protect these important routines by sharing my needs with those around me. Routines such as these have been the key to gaining back my confidence and building self-esteem after my childhood experiences.

Another part of our brain, the cerebral cortex—responsible for the rewiring of our reptilian brain—is the most developed part of the brain, making way for our consciousness, decision making, creativity, objective analysis, and choice of outlook or perspective on any given situation. Our cerebral cortex is what gives us the ability to take a step back after experiencing a powerful emotional trigger and assess the situation. In choosing to take a step back and view a difficult situation with perspective and mindfulness—especially in our most triggered moments—we can begin to address any false beliefs and residual fears we've been operating under as if on autopilot for so long.

At times it may seem like our emotional responses are out of our control. What we may fail to realize is each time a familiar negative feeling is triggered, it's an opportunity to rewire our primitive brain memories. At those times, if we take a moment to do a mindful activity in a safe space and allow ourselves to feel rather than push the feeling away, we will start to see and understand the root of that difficult feeling and examine it from all sides. There's nothing wrong with seeking comfort from others, but we also need to have the tools to handle our strong emotions on our own as well. In an effort to build our personal resilience, mindful activity is a productive strategy for developing the independence to handle difficult feelings on our own, and also provides an opportunity to give ourselves the compassionate understanding we crave from others. Then we can communicate what we're feeling with those we love, rather than just reacting, pointing fingers, or going into emotional shutdown. The trick is to allow the feelings to be as they are, by quieting the mind and observing without self-criticism, avoidance, or distraction. Over time, through self-reflection we can gain insight into how our primitive brain's beliefs and fears are driving the feelings and behaviors we want to change so desperately.

In summary, our bad habits and fears are like Bonnie and Clyde. They work very well together and reinforce each other. Most of our eating habits and stress management techniques have been reinforced through repetition over many, many years, so they are understandably challenging to change even to the slightest degree. However, the good news is, because our brain and gut biome are both malleable and ever changing—as long as we can overcome any initial fear of committing to change—the possibilities go far beyond what you previously could have ever imagined for your body's physical and emotional well-being. Once you've fully committed to addressing the health of your gut, you can start to set clear goals on how you are going to do this by practicing preparing foods that rebalance your gut microbiome and managing your stress in a whole new way. Remember, your nervous system (managed by your response to stressful situations) is driving your inner microbial community's diversity and makeup to the same degree that your microbial flora (directed by diet and routine) is communicating with your nervous system. Once you have clear goals such as cutting out sugar, introducing more mindful activities into your day, learning how to make tasty sauerkraut, investing in a hearty probiotic and/or prebiotic green drink, and/or beginning to include other fermented products in your daily diet, this is when the true transformation begins. Your actions begin to line up with your goals, and your sense of self-worth will soar.

Fear of change will always be present in our lives to some degree, but our job is to *prove it wrong* by constantly challenging our assumptions. Pursuing the life and health we desire may feel as though we're walking across a tightrope suspended high in the air, and we often forget that we need to take it one step at a time and possibly just start with a bar placed right on the ground to practice our balance. All expert tightrope walkers practiced on a tightrope just one foot from the ground for years before attempting one twenty or thirty feet up. Simply acknowledging your microbial community's presence on this journey with you is the first step onto your own internal tightrope, no matter what height it may be at. If you keep asking, over time you will better learn how to distinguish which cravings are coming from unhealthy microbes rooted in fear of their own survival, and which are from beneficial strains guiding you toward real possibility.

FINDING A NEW PERSPECTIVE

When you're at the supermarket and craving a snack, do you sometimes hear an inner voice telling you to buy that container of fresh local blueberries? If the blueberries cost four dollars more than a bag of chips, do you listen to your fear of finances or to your authentic truth? Situations like this challenge us to prove to ourselves how much we truly value our microbial health and our body—the single most important thing we have to take care of in this world. If we are not taking care of ourselves on a regular basis, it's easy to grow resentful. We may not be as present or loving toward our children and family, or even around, as long as we would like to be. Can we even place a dollar value on our energy levels, overall mood, pain levels, and health? How much time and money do we spend perfecting our home, our car, and necessities for our kids so we can create a comfortable, healthy environment to live in? Now it's time to demonstrate your self-worth through how you spend your valuable time and money buying and preparing food and creating habits that will sustain and keep you strong through any challenges that might come your way.

Back in college, before moving to Oregon in search of a new way of living, my priorities were a mess. When I would finally break away for "me time," I'd opt for retail therapy and splurge on clothes, trying to find styles that made me feel thinner and prettier. The irony was that even as I was spending money on clothes, I was so cheap about my diet that I continued eating foods that were processed, refined, and easy to obtain—products that were actually making me gain weight and feel unattractive. Once I started splurging a little extra on healthy, wholesome foods like organic farmer's market veggies, fresh-pressed green juices, organic berries, and whole-fat antibiotic-free yogurt, I actually started to feel better about my body. I didn't need new clothes to build my confidence or try to hide imperfections. Without the added bloat after eating, I felt comfortable and attractive in anything I was wearing.

Let's try to find a new perspective right now. Close your eyes and try to imagine each meal as an opportunity—not a chore or a dreaded land mine of temptation—but a real opportunity to give your healthy microbial community what it deserves—something nourishing, satisfying, and delicious. This is your chance to provide yourself with all the essential nutrients you need to feel energized, alert, confident in your skin, and satisfied until the next meal; a way to give vitamins to your skin and hair to make them shine, and provide wholesome, fiber-filled veggies to your intestines to build healthy bacteria and support your immune system and metabolism. You have a chance to choose something that will sustain your energy and focus for another four to five hours and prevent cravings for unhealthy, nutrient-poor snacks. If you haven't already, take a moment now to imagine how approaching a meal simply with this new intention might change the outlook of your current eating choices. Jot down in a journal what comes into your mind and imagination when you ask yourself these questions: Do you see yourself going to a local farmer's market and buying bundles of juicy fruits or fresh, dewy leafy greens? What sort of foods do you imagine yourself preparing and eating? Maybe you imagine yourself coming home from work and feeling excited and motivated to cook a homemade dinner rather than microwaving leftovers. What is on your plate as you sit down to dinner? Whatever image you see, soak it in and then write it down so you don't forget!

· Yogurt + berries   · Chia seeds   · Chick pea wraps
· Veggie sandwiches + hummus   · Tofu (shredded)   · tuna ☺

CHANGING MIND-SETS CHANGES HABITS

Valuing our mental and physical health goes beyond avoiding sugary, processed, and refined foods. Changing our habits around sugar requires a change in mind-set from autopilot to creative intention in every area of our life. In addition to changing your diet, you're being called to be more creative and in tune with the way you observe yourself and the world around you. Maybe you look forward to going out to eat every day at work because it allows you a break from the office, but there is only fast food available nearby. Looking mindfully at this situation, how can you get a break from the office each day without eating out? Maybe you schedule a walk in the middle of your day, whether it's for lunch, coffee, tea, or just some down time, and find you're getting double the benefits—a boost of energy from your walk and time for mindfulness practice. Maybe you decide to demonstrate your self-worth and appreciation by prioritizing your sleep schedule every night. Or maybe you feel the call to get up fifteen minutes earlier every morning to meditate, and discover that you feel more rested and clear-minded after your meditation than if you had slept that extra fifteen minutes. Tell others in your life about your new intentions to get their support. Ask them to hold you accountable. You don't have to do this alone.

It's time to give up all your usual excuses for why you don't have the health or the life you desire. Remember that you are composed of billions of little microbes that are constantly in flux. In fact, substantial changes happen to your microbiome with every single meal you eat! This affords endless possibilities not only for your health, energy levels, and metabolism, but also for your mood, your life, and your relationships. You have the capacity to transform your gut, your health, and your happiness from the inside out. This can be a reality that *you* create for yourself. After all, you are the biggest expert on your body and responsible for all that it does. Ultimately, you are the only one qualified to do what it takes to overcome any obstacles that stand in your way.

Maybe just the thought of listening to your internal gut wisdom and choosing the right course of action brings about a whole host of insecurities and doubts. This novel approach doesn't mean you won't make mistakes along the way. No one's perfect. But finding your inner voice, trusting it, and following it will guide you toward outcomes you only ever dreamed were possible. It all starts with understanding your own body's signals and trusting your own judgment on how to respond.

SETTING YOUR INTENTION

I hope you're ready, because at this point in the book it's time for you to set your new intentions around eating. Maybe up until now your intention has been to learn how to banish your sugar addiction, or to start balancing your blood sugar so you can lose weight. I'm going to ask you to dream bigger! For example, when you set your intention around diet to completely cleanse your body, balance blood sugar instability, and detox everything toxic you're holding on to, your life will change to accommodate that new mind-set in powerful ways.

Take a break right now, grab a piece of paper, and write down all the changes you want to see in your body, your health, and your life. Focus on *what* you want to see change; don't worry about the *how* quite yet. Write down every little change you desire, no matter how big or how small. If you feel you don't have the foundation to accomplish your larger goals, break them down into smaller goals leading up to larger ones. Your list could be half a page, a whole page, or multiple pages long. The more you write, the better!

- I want to sleep better
- I want to eat foods that fuel me.
  - ↳ heathy vegetables
  - ↳ No meat
  - ↳ No fast food
- Spend less money on take out
- Get stronger for volleyball, running, hikes, etc
- Feel more mobile + flexible
- Experience less body aches, sores + pains
- Read more books, more mentaling stimulating activities
- Practice more yoga, breathing exercises, meditation.
- I'm happy with my weight, but I'd love to be a little leaner, more toned.

· 3 ·

A Secret Microbial Garden

All Disease begins in the gut.

—Hippocrates, the Father of Medicine

Six months after my bathroom epiphany, and despite my best efforts to avoid sugar, I was still struggling more than ever with my sugar cravings. I started researching how *Candida* and other fungi feed off sugar and identified that this was not the only microbe influencing my cravings, mood, and digestion. Our gut has been named our "second brain" due to the 500 million neurons that reside here.[1] There is an entire nervous system that exists entirely in the core of our being—in our gut—called the enteric nervous system (ENS), which contains more neurons than our spinal cord. Within this entity of neurons is a complex network of neurotransmitters and proteins that zap messages between neurons. This incredible circuitry enables it to act independently, giving it a literal "mind of its own" and producing those "gut feelings" that so often go against what our brain, or rational thought, is telling us. Our enteric nervous system is possibly more connected to the rest of our body than our brain, given that it is sending 90 percent of the information passing through the primary visceral nerve, the vagus nerve, to the brain—not the other way around. If our gut is so smart, why don't we listen to it more?

Let's go back to the beginning of my journey healing my own gut. At the time my mother, a holistic doctor, mentioned that *Candida* might be a culprit for many of my symptoms, the research behind pathogenic flora causing the types of symptoms I was experiencing was extremely limited. Nine years ago, when I stood looking in my bathroom mirror trying to understand what was happening to my body, scientists had only discovered 200 species of bacteria in the gut. Only in the past few years, however, have they discovered the human body actually contains ten times more microbial cells than blood cells,[2] with estimates of closer to 40,000 bacterial species residing in the human gut.[3] Evidence has been mounting linking our gut flora with inflammation and chronic metabolic and autoimmune diseases. More of the pieces of the microbiome puzzle are starting to click into place.

Now we know for certain there are literally trillions of microscopic, non-human organisms, with over 10,000 different identified microbial species both in the gastrointestinal tract and throughout the body—on our skin and hair, in our ears, within our organs and bloodstream. Each one of these microbes contains a few thousand genes. All this compared to a paltry 20,000 estimated in the human genome—to say you are outnumbered is a massive understatement. While our human genomes may be 99.9 percent the same, our gut microbiome can be 100 percent different. Just as a bird's-eye view of a city gives little to no information about the individual lives of the actual people living down below, as we now dig deeper we are only beginning to scratch the surface of understanding the intricate yet vital roles our gut micro-bugs play out in their immediate environment, our bodies. For example, there are over 5,000 separate species of bacteria living in our colon alone. Our immune system and metabolism literally depend on these guys to do their work. Scientists are coming to understand that the makeup of our microbiome as a whole often determines whether pathogens in the gut are kept at bay, or cause disease.

There are three classes of microbes in our intestine: commensal (healthy), symbiotic (neutral), and pathogenic (unhealthy).[4] Most experts believe the average healthy mix of microbes is about 85 percent healthy/neutral and 15 percent unhealthy.[5] This ideal composition includes a healthy majority of microbes trained and poised to defend against antigens. The commensal, or healthy flora, that support our digestion and feed on digested fiber and plants include probiotics like *Lactobacillus acidophilus* and *Saccharomyces boulardii*, to name a few. Then there are the pathogenic microbes we need to keep in check, such as the fungus *Candida albicans*, *Clostridium difficile*, and *Proteus mirabilis*. Women are typically very familiar with the *Candida albicans* fungus, as an overgrowth of *Candida* can cause vaginal yeast infections and urinary tract infections in females.[6]

Let's return to the river ecosystem metaphor raised in the previous chapter, where the rapid overgrowth of one invasive species of underwater fern can threaten the survival of other underwater plants as it conquers more and more territory. Soon healthy fish and bacteria—also a part of this delicate ecosystem reliant on sunlight and now blocked by the tentacles of the large fern overgrowth—start to die off. In a similar way, if an imbalance exists in our microbiome, it can cause a ripple effect, resulting in diminished beneficial flora that can manifest itself in many different ways throughout the entire ecosystem of the human body. An imbalance of the microflora in our bodies can impact our blood cells, immune cells, nutrient storage, organs, hormones, and neurotransmitters like dopamine, serotonin, cortisol, and other chemicals that help us balance our mood and manage stress.[7]

How do you know if you have bad or imbalanced gut bacteria? The symptoms that can accompany either a general imbalance or insufficiency of beneficial flora are quite diverse; however, there are a few general symptoms you can look for. One of the most common signs of overgrowth and/or lack of diversity is bloating. When an overgrowth of bacteria or fungi is exposed to high-carbohydrate foods in your diet in the large intestine, they will ferment and produce excessive gas, which can also cause intestinal pain and belching and lead to reflux from the increased pressure in the intestinal tract.[8] Constipation and diarrhea are also common symptoms to watch for, with constipation being a leading cause of methane breath production, which is a common cause of "bad breath."[9] If you experience a small amount of largely odorless gas from time to time, that is considered completely normal; however, if you are experiencing gas, bad breath, painful flatulence, and/or reflux on an everyday basis, then something is likely awry. It's also possible to have an imbalance in the gut microbiome and *not* experience any obvious symptoms of this nature. It can manifest in other ways such as anxiety, fibromyalgia, Crohn's disease, metabolic syndrome, colon cancer, and autism, among many other diseases.[10]

A CASE FOR *MORE* MICROBES

Given our culture's obsession with antibacterial soaps, sprays, and cleaners, it may come as a shock to hear that the vast majority of the microbes in and around us, especially outdoors in nature, are actually critical to maintaining our health. These tiny bugs help us fight off viruses and pathogens, digest our fruits and vegetables, extract the vitamins and minerals from our food, and process glucose that our cells use for energy. They help regulate our metabolism, build critical hormones and vitamins to keep our nervous system and mood in check, and play a large role in determining how our genes are expressed—given the fact that these microbes make up over 99 percent of the genetic material in our bodies.[11] Our parents' genetics, which define our unique human genome, account for less than 1 percent of our total genes. While this 1 percent may set up the possibility of developing disease based on family genes, an even smaller number of those with a genetic marker for a specific disease will actually develop that disease. The chances of developing a disease based on familial genetics alone is by no means a foregone conclusion. Why do some with a genetic marker for certain illnesses get sick and others don't?

Science is increasingly looking to our microbiome and a lack of microbial diversity found there. If we share the same environment growing up with our parents—the same foods, the same lifestyle, and similar medications—we're basically reproducing a very similar microbiome composition, and it makes sense that we are likely to develop the same health problems. However, if we choose to take a different path, we can drastically differentiate our microbiome, repopulating our body with healthy, life-giving flora. Our changed microbiome then reduces our chances of having the same health problems as our relatives.

Our gut flora is made up of a variety of immune cells lining the intestine, called the mucosal immune system. This system comprises more than 75 percent of the immune system, acting as the first line of defense when bad bacteria dare to enter. We spoke earlier of how the majority of genes in our body are microbial. Well, the same is true for the majority of the cells in our body. That's because less than 50 percent of all the cells in our body are actually, well, human![12] The remaining cells are bacteria, fungi, and other microbes. These gut bugs making up our mucosal immune system are constantly overseeing the gut environment in addition to the surfaces of the body most vulnerable to pathogens. Our lungs, nose, eyes, mouth, ears, and throat all have direct exposure to the outside environment. This frontier is where healthy bacteria should be allowed entry into the body and bad bacteria should be stopped. The health and diversity of our microbiome is a key determinant of what transpires on this frontier when there is contact with the outside environment.

Perhaps even more importantly, the microbes in our gut break down all the plant fiber we eat—fruits, vegetables, and all other nutrient-dense plants—so that we can absorb the vitamins and minerals. Healthy gut bugs also produce nutrients like vitamin K, serotonin, and other essential hormones, along with the neurotransmitters we rely on to function optimally. If we don't have a strong microbiome, our body may develop vitamin and mineral deficiencies and subsequently won't have the building blocks to make all the essential hormones and neurotransmitters we rely so heavily on to stay and feel healthy. Our microbes regulate the way calories are extracted from food, and therefore also regulate metabolism, appetite, and food cravings. In some studies where microbiota from lean people were transplanted into obese subjects, those previously overweight individuals not only lost weight, but experienced personality changes as well.[13] These changes were observed because a new set of genes have literally been transferred into their bodies!

Our mucosal immune system performs its protective feat in two ways. First, it initiates a pro-inflammatory response when reacting to a threat. Then it follows up with an anti-inflammatory response once the threat has receded.[14] When there is abundant diversity in the mucosal immune system, our microflora helps us achieve a balance between these two responses. However, if the pro-inflammatory response happens too often, often due to lack of the beneficial microbes needed to restore the balance, then inflammation and unhealthy microbes can overrun the intestine. In a process akin to mixing ingredients to bake bread, our bodies will be healthy to the extent that the mixture of healthy, neutral, and unhealthy microbes in our intestines are in the correct ratio—but you also need the right temperature. If things start to get too hot, with inflammation running out of control, the chance of the metaphorical microbial batter turning disease-ridden skyrockets. This is a somewhat over-simplified representation of what happens behind the scenes of inflammatory bowel disease (IBD), such as Crohn's disease and ulcerative colitis, when inflammation in the gut starts to run rampant.

Researchers at the California Institute of Technology have estimated that the recent sevenfold increase in rates of autoimmune disorders including Crohn's disease, type 1 diabetes, and multiple sclerosis is due to the lack of beneficial microbes in our gut.[15] Unbalanced gut flora have also been linked to a host of diseases ranging from autism and depression to autoimmune conditions such as Hashimoto's disease, other inflammatory bowel diseases, and chronic fatigue syndrome. At the time I was struggling with my own early warning signs of health problems, my doctors did not even consider whether microbiome activity could be culpable, because research findings on the microbiome had not been widely disseminated. Even today, a medical paradigm that includes a microbiome health perspective has yet to become integrated into medical school training. Training remains largely focused on treating the presenting symptoms directly, rather than possible root causes.

What are some of the major reasons for a lack of diversity of the microbes populating our gut and the resulting overgrowth of pathogenic microbes in the body? There are a number of factors, including diet, stress, certain medications such as antibiotics, nonsteroidal anti-inflammatory drugs (NSAIDs), birth control pills, antibacterial soaps and sprays, and even whether we were born via cesarean delivery or were bottle- versus breast-fed. An overgrowth of *Clostridium difficile* is most common following a regimen of broad-spectrum antibiotics and can lead to chronic, long-term loose stools and excessive watery, diarrhea-like stools.[16] In more severe cases a *Clostridium difficile* overgrowth can become an infection causing abdominal cramping and severe pain, watery diarrhea throughout the day, fever, nausea, and loss of appetite. *Proteus mirabilis* overgrowth is commonly known to cause urinary tract infections; however, the majority of urinary tract infections are due to *E. coli* overgrowth.

Until recently, you would only know if you had an overgrowth of pathogenic flora if you developed a more commonly known severe infection as a result. But many people suffered from mild overgrowth of pathogenic flora for years without treatment because doctors couldn't detect these mild cases with the standard tests available, or they wouldn't know to test for them without an accompanying fever. Even if doctors did test for mild cases of pathogenic overgrowth, the only treatment at their disposal may be yet another round of antibiotics! Only in recent years are innovative companies like Genova Diagnostics developing more comprehensive stool tests that many holistic health practitioners are now using. These tests provide a score reflecting the total number of an individual patient's commensal (beneficial) bacteria that are out of normal range so a probiotic containing the specific strains missing or lacking can be prescribed. Probiotic supplements are not a fix-all, but they are a great first step, along with dietary changes, to restoring balance to our delicate micro-ecosystem. Even these tests and supplemental treatments are still in their early days, so our strongest recourse is to take a look at everything, from our diet to our cravings to our lifestyle, and start to make little changes here and there.

SAVE YOUR ENDANGERED SPECIES!

With all the attention we give to the diminishing biodiversity on our planet, there is an even more important ecological reality that we are not giving enough attention to. The most important endangered species we need to focus our attention on saving are the ones facing extinction in our own internal ecosystem.

I don't know if I would call myself an avid environmentalist per se, but I do make considerable efforts to reduce garbage waste in our home through composting and recycling, using reusable bags when shopping, and trying not to leave a carbon footprint by taking the train to work and walking to the store whenever I can. I try to be mindful not to waste our planet's precious resources for the sake of convenience. Just as we might think about our planet as our only home and strive to make efforts not to contribute to the decimation of its vast species of flora and fauna for the sake of our own convenience, we must treat our body with the same respect. Our bodies are quite literally the first and only home we have. As a civilized species in the Western Hemisphere, with chlorinated running water and temperature-controlled homes, gyms, and offices—giving us little reason to ever go outside, we are getting sicker and sicker due to the trillions of beneficial bacterial species dying off every day.

In a multinational study published in 2013, scientists studied the number of genes in the microbiome of 169 obese Danish individuals and 123 Danish individuals with a healthy weight. They realized that the Danish population could be broken into two main groups based on the diversity of microbes in their gut, or "bacterial richness," as they called it.[17] Not surprisingly, the group that had very low diversity in their microbes consisted of the overweight and obese individuals. This group had much higher insulin resistance and inflammation compared to the leaner group. High insulin resistance and greater inflammation constitute two main factors creating a perfect metabolic storm for weight gain and chronic conditions such as type 2 diabetes, cardiovascular and liver diseases, and cancer. Those with a healthier microbiome had bacterial genes favoring creation of short-chain fatty acids, which have been shown to reduce the risk of inflammatory diseases, type 2 diabetes, obesity, heart disease, and other conditions. Our bacterial genes are responsible for making these crucial short-chain fatty acids within our bodies, thus protecting us from illness and maintaining our health.[18]

It would be an easier problem to solve if we could point to one change in our diet or environment in the last one hundred years that is responsible for the reduction in the bacterial diversity we are seeing lately, leading to the rise in chronic illness. However, it's not that simple. Due to a close tie with our enteric nervous system, literally everything we come in contact with affects our microbiome—including every positive or fearful thought we have. Our body's stress response has a huge impact on our digestion and the health of our microbiome, and this "gut-brain axis" explains why social or psychological stress can also affect our overall health and the development of illness, which we'll get into later.

However, there are a few major changes in our external environment in the last one hundred years responsible for the lack of biodiversity in our intestines. These include an increase of sugar and hybridized refined wheat in our diet, an increase in antibiotic usage and over-sanitation practices, and a decrease in organic, fermented food consumption made possible by the advent of refrigeration in the 1930s. Most conventionally raised meats these days are treated with broad-spectrum antibiotics, which is another way antibiotics get into our system and destroy many strains of our healthy flora. Put simply, wheat, sugar—including "natural sugars" such as lactose and fructose, and meat and dairy products from conventionally raised animals reduce the diversity and quantity of healthy microflora in our gut, causing gut dysbiosis.[19]

There may not be much we can do about the fact that much of the conventional produce found in supermarkets these days has been treated with herbicides and is therefore lacking in beneficial microbes. But we can buy local and organic produce whenever possible and seek out Community Supported Agriculture (CSA) opportunities in our area. We may no longer live in homes with dirt floors, which provided us with exposure to microbe-rich dirt all day long, giving us the microbes we needed for immunity from a young age to all sorts of bacterial species found in our environment. But we can avoid overuse of antibacterial soaps and sprays, chemical cleaners, and hand sanitizers in our own homes—seeking instead cleaners made with essential oils and other natural ingredients. Additionally, opening our windows, weather permitting, to allow a fresh gust of healthy microbes into our home has merit. We may no longer need to ferment and jar foods to survive the winter, but we can still make and buy fermented foods like sauerkraut or kimchi or yogurt. We may not need to make our own herbal iced or hot tea elixirs, because we can walk into any corner store and choose from a pre-bottled sugar-sweetened tea, but our gut biome would prefer if we made our own batch at home from organic, herbal, and maybe even medicinal tea sweetened with raw honey or stevia. Carrying these home-brewed drinks in a glass or insulated stainless steel water bottle avoids exposure to the harmful microbe-killing chemicals found in plastics used in both canned and bottled drinks. Most of us no longer forage for nutritious, medicinal bitter greens to treat common ailments in today's modern day, but we can still grow an herb garden in our own backyard. We can order a supplemental powder of microgreens to nourish our beneficial flora and support our immune system, especially in the winter when local organic leafy greens like bok choy, mesclun greens, and spinach are not as readily available. For those of us interested in harvesting prebiotics in our own gardens, kale is a hearty winter green that can grow into December in most northern climates, providing nourishment for our biomes throughout the winter.

WESTERN MEDICAL INTERVENTIONS

Antibiotics don't distinguish the good bacteria from the bad in our bodies. In addition to targeting the possible infection or illness, an antibiotic attack on unhealthy bacteria will also decimate our healthy, beneficial bacteria population in its wake. They kill off a lot of the good or commensal bacteria, as well as some neutral bacteria responsible for keeping pathogenic strains at bay. Antibiotics are designed to kill bacteria, not fungi, which is why an overgrowth of *Candida*, a yeast in the fungi family, is common after taking antibiotics. If both probiotics, in the form of fermented foods, and prebiotics, such as greens and fibrous foods, are not introduced back into the gut immediately after taking antibiotics, chances are high that bad fungi like *Candida* will take hold and flourish. For a weak digestive system, either during or immediately following an infection or antibiotic regimen, be sure to ingest plant fiber in the form of soft, well-cooked vegetable soups and/ or blended green smoothies. Raw plant fiber can be taxing on a weak gut lacking the necessary bacteria to break down and digest food and may cause indigestion.

While antibiotics can be useful, and necessary in many circumstances, these medications are often prescribed to treat ailments like the common cold and other minor conditions or viruses, against which they are useless. If antibiotics are ever recommended by a physician without a clear bacterial test confirming the infection, take precaution. Chances are high the illness could be viral and won't even respond to antibiotics; if that's the case, the devastation on your gut flora would be for nothing. Research has shown that even a typical five-day course of a common antibiotic, ciprofloxin, can kill off one-third of our gut microbiome, leaving an imbalance of bacteria and fungi and reduced biodiversity in the gut—taking up to two years for the gut to recover after treatment.[20]

Although antibiotics may be necessary to fight off serious bacterial infections, they are often given to newborns and young infants at the critical stage of developing their microbiome, where killing off a large portion of these essential microbes can cause permanent harm to the immune system. In rare cases, especially in low-birth-weight infants, excessive antibiotic usage can be deadly.[21] Remember how I mentioned our microbiome and its diversity largely affects our metabolism? Numerous well-documented studies on the long-term ramifications of overuse of antibiotics during infancy show that babies given broad-spectrum antibiotics before age two also have a higher chance of becoming obese during childhood and adulthood.[22, 23]

Being born by cesarean delivery, rather than vaginal birth, also creates a predisposition to a weakened microbiome due to lack of exposure to the essential microflora the baby comes in contact with on the way out of the birth canal. Alternatively, being breast-fed strengthens the microbiome by providing healthy flora through breast milk, establishing increased biodiversity from birth.

If a course of antibiotics is necessary, taking probiotics can help restore some balance in your microbiome. In most cases, every course of antibiotics creates permanent negative alterations in the composition of healthy bacteria, leaving precious real estate in your intestine up for grabs and allowing pathogenic bacteria and fungi, such as *Candida* and *Clostridium difficile*, to take ownership and flourish.[24, 25] *Candida*, in turn, is a type of yeast that lives off excess glucose and sugar from our diet. A history of antibiotic usage combined with regular feeding of a sugar craving is the perfect cocktail for a long-term disrupted microbiome, as was the case for me.[26]

I had chronic ear infections as a baby in an era where it was largely unknown how to prevent or treat ear infections naturally. I was prescribed broad-spectrum antibiotics over and over again between the ages of two and five, when my microbiome was in a vulnerable stage of development. Today, as a mother myself I take a preventative approach by using all-natural antibacterial ear drops, such as garlic mullein herbal tinctures, in my daughter's ears at the first sign of any cold or virus to prevent ear infections from forming. Despite my daughter having inherited her mother's earlobes, this natural approach so far has prevented a single ear infection from developing. I also take further measures to regularly introduce new microbes through probiotics to her developing immune system. When she was a baby I pureed all her baby food at home using organic and local (whenever possible) fruits and vegetables. I also encourage her to crawl and roll around in the dirt on a regular basis and routinely add a probiotic green powder into her bottle. We live in a house built in the 1920s, so lead and dirt quality has always been a concern for us. We make sure she plays far away from any dirt that would have direct contact with our house. We primarily encourage her to play in the garden beds and raised vegetable beds in our yard, which are free of any chemicals or pesticides. We personally filled our garden beds with organic mulch and homemade compost, so we know this dirt is safe for her to play in.

With a young toddler at home, I know how difficult it can be to avoid taking antibiotic medications yourself or giving them to your young child at some point. That's why, should you need to take antibiotics yourself or give them to your child, it's so important to make up for a loss in biodiversity by providing a consistent variety of foods and supplements that contain healthy probiotics and prebiotics for at least three to six months after taking antibiotics—ideally incorporating them into your family's everyday diet for life.

Other medications that can have a detrimental effect on our gut flora are nonsteroidal anti-inflammatory drugs (NSAIDs) and hormones such as birth control pills and steroids. Many more-integrative-minded physicians steer people away from overuse of NSAIDs, such as naproxen-sodium (Aleve), aspirin, and ibuprofen (Advil) due to evidence showing how damaging they are to our intestines and the gut lining.[27] Yet for many people these medications are still go-to household therapies we consider "safe." Because of the popularity of these drugs, high amounts are passed through sewers into groundwater, which then shows up in drinking water. It can be almost impossible to avoid them. In our home we use a $200 countertop charcoal- and sediment-based gravity-powered filtration system to filter out and mineralize our water, so we can hydrate with clean, mineral-rich water. It's a win-win given that our biome loves minerals too.

PATHOGENIC FLORA

If the microbial environment in the intestine gets disrupted by stress, antibiotics, medications, sugar and other processed foods, or a probiotic- or prebiotic-deficient diet—more often than not, a combination of these factors—then opportunistic flora start to grow uninhibited. Two of the most common conditions of overgrowth to watch out for are *Candida* (fungi overgrowth) and small intestinal bacterial overgrowth, also called SIBO. Anytime the diversity in healthy microbes in the gut flora diminishes is a prime opportunity for one or more pathogenic species to grow unencumbered.

The philosophy of treating the root cause of an illness, rather than the presenting symptoms alone—so fundamental to integrative healing modalities—is the approach I take both with my own health and in my health coaching practice. Similar to the earlier river ecosystem analogy, when a root condition is not addressed, even something as simple as a food allergy initiating a pro-inflammatory response in the intestines, or an overgrowth of fungi or bacteria, for example, can have a ripple effect throughout the body and cause other symptoms to manifest. Small amounts of non-commensal, or unhealthy, bacteria and fungi normally reside in our intestinal tract. As in any natural environment, a plant is only identified as a "weed" once that plant starts to kill off other species and take over. A small amount of *Candida albicans*, a type of yeast in the fungi family, is a normal part of the diverse makeup of our internal ecosystem and generally does not cause any harm—as long as it is kept at bay by other beneficial microbes. This type of flora doesn't do all the wonderful things our healthy microbes do for us and belongs to the family of pathogenic microbes, because when it starts to dominate internal space, it can cause harm. Much like a pesky weed in your garden, the overgrowth of *Candida albicans* could lead to blood sugar imbalances,[28] a weakened immune system,[29] and yeast infections and urinary tract infections,[30] as well as have a negative impact on the liver, kidneys, and spleen.[31] Our liver and kidneys are affected because *Candida albicans* produces an increase in the exotoxins that our liver and kidneys are responsible for cleaning out of our blood.[32] If the internal environment becomes ideal for proliferation of *Candida albicans*, it will begin to grow and spread throughout the intestine and sometimes even into the bloodstream.[33]

As it turns out, the diet and culture in the United States creates the ideal conditions for an overgrowth of *Candida*. In fact, candida is an extremely common condition, affecting 70 percent of the U.S. population, according to molecular biologists at Rice University.[34] Julia Koehler, a Harvard University fellow in infectious disease, found that candida is the predominant fungal infection behind human disease, making it a largely unknown health epidemic.[35] Perhaps by no coincidence, all our favorite sweet foods happen to be the favorite food of this particular strain of microscopic fungi, literally feeding this internal weed as it starts to overrun the healthy cornucopia of flora and fauna in our intestines.

When this particular pathogenic flora starts to become systemic, it becomes a much larger problem. In people whose immune systems are already weakened by serious illness or old age, *Candida* in the bloodstream can become the actual cause of death, as is often the case in hospital settings where patients are also being treated heavily with antibiotics.[36] Based on research published in the *Journal of the German Society of Dermatology*, the overgrowth of the particular strain *Candida albicans* may be responsible for 50 to 90 percent of candida infections as well as being the root of many other chronic diseases.[37] More often, however, an overgrowth is not life-threatening and may not yet be contributing to chronic illness, but may be leading to a myriad of mysterious symptoms such as yeast infections, urinary tract infections, a weakened immune system, bloat after eating, newfound sensitivies to common foods, indigestion, minor vitamin deficiencies, infections, acne and skin rashes, dizziness, anxiety, weight gain, and fatigue.[38] As you may recall, the mysterious health problems I suffered from included many of these exact symptoms—including, of course, an insatiable sweet tooth.

Small intestinal bacterial overgrowth (SIBO) needs to be treated with a similar diet and herbal treatments as a *Candida* overgrowth. Because it is bacterial, the most common medical treatment for this condition is in fact to take *more* antibiotics! However, studies have shown herbal antimicrobials to be just as effective as antibiotics, and in some cases more effective, in the treatment of this condition. One study showed that 46 percent of the patients treated with herbal antimicrobials were successfully treated while only 34 percent were free of SIBO after taking the leading antibiotic Rifaximin.[39] This study also showed antimicrobial herbs to be extremely effective in getting rid of SIBO (57 percent) even after an unsuccessful course of antibiotics. Researchers in the study used herbal supplements that contain a powerful combination of herbal antimicrobials including, but not limited to, oregano, thyme, sage, lemon balm, Oregon grape, ginger rhizome, Chinese licorice root, Chinese rhubarb root, and pau d'arco bark.

SUGAR PARTY IN YOUR GUT

Bread bakers know that yeast grows best in warm, moist places with sugar to eat. As an opportunistic yeast and member of the fungi family,[40] *Candida* thrives where there is consistently high glucose, in a hypoglycemic environment.[41] Yeast feeds on sugar and high-glycemic foods. Juice, cookies, bread, milk, candy, and alcohol are some of its favorite foods. The more consistently we have extra glucose floating around, the more *Candida* will grow and thrive. Such an environment in turn will disrupt blood sugar equilibrium even more, making us crave sweets and feel those hunger pangs stronger and more often, creating a dangerous cycle that can be hard to break. In a study testing diabetic patients for the presence of oral yeasts, researchers found *Candida albicans* to be the primary yeast (60 percent) among a variety of pathogenic yeasts including *Candida tropicalis, Candida krusei, Candida guilliermondii, Candida parapsilosis,* and *Toruloposis candida,* and 41 percent of the diabetic patients tested had some form of candida. Their blood glucose level at the time of testing was the biggest causal factor of whether the diabetic patients had *Candida* overgrowth or not.[42]

Given that alcohol is created through a fermentation process involving yeast and sugar—the two ingredients that *Candida* loves best, alcohol consumption can particularly exacerbate *Candida* overgrowth as well. Of course, diet alone is not the only catalyst for *Candida* overgrowth. As we discussed earlier, many other factors like medications, stress, and antibiotics play important roles in weakening the biodiversity of our gut flora. Diet, however, often determines which types of species grow back, and without reintroducing beneficial bacteria quickly, the fungi left in the aftermath of the antibiotic or stressful episode will have nothing to inhibit their growth.

Was my biological predisposition to blood sugar problems the cause of my sugar cravings and the trigger for *Candida*? Was *Candida* causing me to be more susceptible to blood sugar imbalance? Or was *Candida* simply messing with my blood sugar by literally eating all the excess glucose in my blood and causing my blood sugar to drop? Most likely all three scenarios were in play. However, the microbiome I developed when I was young, from exposure to my parent's microbiome and from living in a similar way to my parents, is likely a cause of my predisposition to blood sugar imbalance. Coupled with the many frequent rounds of antibiotics I took as a child, which killed off a lot of my healthy bacteria, this created the right environment for fungi such as *Candida* to feed off my excess blood sugar and cause further blood sugar imbalance that left me starving and craving more sugar.

Researchers at the University of California found that *Candida* affects blood sugar in other ways as well, by making an enzyme called aspartyl protease, or SAP, which works by destroying the receptor sites on cells, preventing glucose from entering to fuel cells.[43] In effect, you could have just eaten a few hours ago and still be starving and tired because much of the glucose you ate didn't even make it into your cells to produce energy. This additional process can be a major challenge to our blood sugar levels. In this case glucose levels rise abnormally high because they are not being allowed entry into vital cells that make up our tissues and organs, and they're left floating around instead, causing a spike in blood sugar and a further feast for *Candida*. These greedy microbes want all the glucose for themselves! This feeding frenzy can in turn stimulate a blood sugar pendulum swing that can lead to additional sugar cravings and increased *Candida* growth.

Once there is an overgrowth of these sugar-loving microbes in your intestine, they will consume blood sugar quickly, you may be left hungry or craving sugar not long after a meal. At the height of my health problems, my blood sugar would drop within hours of a meal. I became ravenously hungry, craving anything that could restore my blood sugar level the quickest. Sugar, refined carbs, and other processed foods fit the bill. In short, my pathogenic flora began running the show. I was craving more and more sugar, which was slowing down my metabolism and increasing my appetite.[44] On the other hand, a balanced microbiome reduces cravings for unhealthy foods, revs up our metabolism, and balances blood sugar so we don't get quite so hungry nearly as often.

After starting my gut detox regimen, the first step I took was to adopt a strict diet of avoiding foods high in sugar and refined grains. I began eating lots of prebiotic foods such as high-fiber cruciferous vegetables and leafy greens like cabbage, broccoli, fresh herbs, kale, rainbow and Swiss chard, spinach, and dandelion greens, and began including raw fermented foods in my diet on a daily basis. I chose a probiotic supplement containing *lactobacillus, saccharomyces*, and *bifidobacterium*, three powerful strains of healthy bacteria to help rebuild an environment where my healthy microflora could thrive. *Lactobacilli*—found in cultured yogurt, cheese, kefir, raw sauerkraut, kimchi, and pickles—are some of the easiest probiotics to supplement in your diet. I've created a similar regimen with my health coaching clients today.

Elizabeth came to me complaining of fatigue, foggy thinking, bloat after eating, anxiety, and recent weight gain. Her symptoms weren't severe enough to be diagnosable by a physician, yet she was sure something was out of whack. As a mother of two, she admitted she would often grab bread and other baked goods when she was hungry and on-the-go with her kids. She was also an avid baker and loved eating fresh-baked goods. Yet her energy levels seemed to be draining more every day, and she was starting to lose faith in her ability to keep up with the demands of being a full-time mom. At my direction she cleaned out her kitchen of sugar and refined grains, including all gluten, and started adding in probiotics and prebiotics regularly. She introduced store-bought and homemade raw sauerkraut, and a probiotic supplement with eight different strains of healthy flora, as well as a green smoothie made with kale, spinach, and spirulina powder blended with ripe banana and apple for breakfast. Things turned around for her in just a couple of months. She came back to me a new woman two months after our initial consultation. "Not only have all my symptoms disappeared, but I'm even sleeping better, am more calm and less anxious than I can remember feeling since before I became a mother and started losing sleep from night feedings," she said. "Plus, I've started to bake breads and muffins with new ingredients like coconut flour, almond flour, and spelt flour, sweetened with applesauce and ripe bananas instead of sugar. They are delicious; even my kids love them."

As mentioned earlier, the symptoms of bacterial overgrowth (SIBO) are very similar to *Candida* (fungi overgrowth). Luckily, the same treatment will work for both, so you don't necessarily need to know which condition of microbial overgrowth you have to start treatment. Diet is a powerful way to alter the gut microbiome and replenish our beneficial flora.[45] As long as we avoid high-glycemic foods such as sugar and refined grains, and add in probiotics and prebiotics, our intestinal flora may be able to recover on their own. Once we're caught in an unhealthy cycle long enough and it starts to become a systemic condition, however, reinforcements will need to be called in to help kill off the overgrowth. Herbal and food-based antifungals and antibacterial tinctures and teas such as garlic, oregano, and pau d'arco, for example, can help reduce the overgrowth of pathogenic fungi or bacteria, while eating probiotic foods like raw sauerkraut and yogurt restores beneficial bacteria to the gut. If you suspect you may have candida or SIBO, see below for a list of common symptoms and my Intestinal Restore Cleanse.

Symptoms Associated with Candida and SIBO

> Fatigue or lethargy
> Depression intermittent with periods of high and intense energy
> Headaches, muscle aches
> Abdominal pain including feeling bloated and gassy
> Indigestion
> Sensitivity to milk or wheat or other food allergies
> Rectal itching
> Constipation and/or diarrhea
> Mouth rashes including "white tongue"
> Bad breath
> Frequent colds
> Respiratory or other infections
> Drowsiness
> Irritability—especially when hungry
> Mood swings
> Premenstrual problems
> Attacks of anxiety or crying
> Insomnia
> Dizziness or loss of balance
> Cold hands or feet and low body temperature
> Hypothyroidism

Eczema
Psoriasis
Chronic hives
Cystitis or interstitial cystitis (painful bladder syndrome).

If you have five or more of these ailments on an occasional basis, there's a good chance you may have a mild form of candida or SIBO. If you have at least five of these symptoms frequently or severely, then you may have a more chronic overgrowth.[46]

Questionnaire

If you suspect you have a fungal or bacterial overgrowth, here is a quick five-minute questionnaire to find out if the symptoms you are experiencing are likely caused by candida or SIBO:

1. Have you at any time in your life taken broad-spectrum antibiotics or other antibacterial medication for respiratory or urinary tract infections, acne, or other health conditions for more than two months or at least three times in a single year? Yes/No
2. Have you taken birth control pills for at least six months? Yes/No
3. Have you ever taken steroids for two weeks or more? Yes/No
4. In the past year, have you had athlete's foot, ringworm, "jock itch," yeast infections, or other fungal infections? Yes/No
5. Do you crave sugar often (every one to two days)? Yes/No

INTESTINAL RESTORE CLEANSE

A pathogenic flora overgrowth can be stubborn to get rid of and a major cause of sugar cravings. If you suspect you suffer from fungal or bacterial overgrowth, it's best to do the following cleanse while reducing sugar and refined carbohydrates in your diet. Personally, I simply did not have the willpower to reduce sugar in my diet without addressing my *Candida* with antifungal herbs simultaneously. This is because when *Candida* is pervasive it requires high blood glucose to live and results in your blood sugar dropping extremely low, which triggers sugar cravings. Addressing your blood sugar swings by completely avoiding refined carbohydrates, eating plenty of healthy fats (nuts, seeds, nut butter, avocados, avocado oil, butter, coconut oil, and olive oil) and replacing refined sugars with natural alternatives and/or keeping sugars under ten grams a day will also further reduce *Candida* overgrowth and sugar cravings.

Taking antifungal herbs, in addition to taking a probiotic, can be necessary to reset your microflora and kill off pathogenic fungi. Whole herbs gently help the body with detoxification and purification, and reduce inflammation in the gut. Certain herbs are very high in minerals and antifungals, which create an environment *Candida* or harmful bacteria cannot survive in. The most powerful natural antifungal herbs for *Candida* and SIBO include oregano, garlic, pau d'arco, black walnut, and cloves. I discovered, through trial and error, that the closer the herb is to its whole plant form the more effective it will be. For example, taking a tincture of these herbs or drinking large quantities of herbal tea steeped for at least twenty minutes is a fresher, more whole form of these herbs compared to most capsules or supplements. Herbal tinctures are concentrated liquid extracts of herbs. The extraction process involves simply letting whole plants sit in alcohol for weeks or months, which allows the medicinal properties to be gently drawn out of the plant without changing the chemical structure of these plant components. If you are pregnant or nursing do not take antimicrobial herbs. Stick to Red Raspberry leaf tea, Ginger tea, and Echinacea tea.

If you are going to take a supplement of an herb, make sure it is of the highest quality. It is important that any capsule contains the highest quality, most potent, herbs. Many of the supplements in the store use diluted or poor-quality ingredients, so be wary and don't waste your money! CandiBactin-AR and Candibactin-BR by the company Metagenics, contain high-quality oregano and thyme oil blended with other herbal extracts. These supplements work just as effectively as antibiotics on treatment of SIBO, according to research.[47] Para-Gard by Integrative Therapeutics is also effective at treating both fungal and bacterial overgrowth. This is one of the recommendations in my Intestinal Restore Cleanse outlined at the end of this section. Metagenics and Integrative Therapeutics perform rigorous testing on all their supplements, which are some of the highest therapeutic- and clinical-grade supplements available. Other well-researched, quality antimicrobial supplements are Dysbiocide and FC Cidal by Biotics Research Laboratories.

Be sure to consult with a trained herbalist or holistic practitioner before taking any of these supplements as they can be much stronger than herbal teas and tinctures and may have minor side effects if taken at a high dose. Activated charcoal will help pull the die-off of harmful microbes out of your intestine and reduce gas and bloating during your cleanse. Both are common side effects of pathogenic microbial die-off and are typically experienced in the first few days of starting antimicrobial herbs. These symptoms should be gone three to five days after starting this cleanse. Activated charcoal must be taken in supplement form, and I recommend Integrative Therapeutics brand. L-Glutamine is a vital amino acid the intestine requires to rebuild and repair from imbalanced microflora. It can also help reduce any diarrhea, gas, and bloat you experience during your cleanse, reduce cravings for sugar and alcohol, and aid in the detoxification process. I recommend an L-Glutamine supplement in this cleanse; however, one to two cups of bone broth is also high in L-Glutamine and can be substituted for this supplement. Finally, probiotics are an essential component in rebalancing your internal microbe environment. Taking a good-quality probiotic will not only help build healthy bacteria and fungi in your gut, but also help with any food sensitivities and poor nutrient absorption that is common among individuals suffering from an imbalance. Check out the refrigerator section at your local health food store for a probiotic supplement that contains at least six strains of living bacteria.

During your cleanse you will be completely avoiding sugar, dairy, wheat, and alcohol. Consume large quantities of cruciferous vegetables including, but not limited to, cauliflower, kale, brussels sprouts, cabbage, bok choy, Swiss chard, broccoli rabe, broccoli, and green leafy vegetables. These types of vegetables help restore minerals to the gut to build back your healthy flora and aid the body's detoxification system. Leafy greens and cruciferous vegetables also support a healthy microbiome and the optimal functioning of the digestive, reproductive, and detoxification systems. Foods that are natural antimicrobials include onions, garlic, and coconut. Ginger is a powerful immune enhancer, supports digestion, and acts as a prokinetic, a substance that stimulates movement within the small intestine. After peeling the skin off fresh ginger root (I scrape it off with a butter knife), you can chop it up and add to any stir-fry or vegetable dish, blend into smoothies, or boil in water for a strong ginger tea. Coconut oil is a potent *Candida* killer and one of the most potent antifungals there is. It contains lauric acid and caprylic acid, which both help prevent *Candida* overgrowth and strengthen your immune system. Onions and garlic both have powerful antifungal properties and help boost the immune system. If you do the double punch—starve the *Candida* while killing them with antifungals and herbs—you can be sure they won't survive.

In addition to these dietary specifications, the three most important elements of the cleanse are taking antimicrobial herbs throughout the day, taking probiotics at least once a day, and drinking lots of water or herbal teas. Water is essential while taking herbs to assist your body with this cleansing or "die-off" process. Within twenty-four hours of starting to take high-quality herbs, your *Candida* or bacterial overgrowth will start to die off; this is when you may experience some gas or bloating. You can assist this process by drinking large quantities of water to support your liver, and by consuming lots of vegetables and high-fiber foods to keep your bowels loose and able to dispose of the dead microbes. Green smoothies are a great way to get up to six servings of fruits and vegetables in one meal.

Most clients I've worked with feel dramatically better within a few weeks on this cleanse, and after only one month have largely restored their microbial balance. However, if you suspect you might suffer from a more chronic over-growth, you may experience a resurgence of symptoms within a few weeks of stopping the herbs and may need to continue for another one to two months.

The key to a successful and quick recovery are the diet changes described throughout this book. Make sure you are eating foods that balance your blood sugar, and include lots of whole unrefined grains and vegetables to feed your healthy gut flora throughout the cleanse. It also is vital to avoid all sugar and refined carbohydrates. Herbs and supplements can help you jump-start this process, but without the dietary changes you will find it hard to sustain long-term health. If you need a sweet fix, better to have some brown rice with raw honey and butter, an apple with peanut butter, or oatmeal with no more than one teaspoon of maple syrup than to eat anything that comes in a box or is a refined form of sugar. A small amount (one teaspoon) of raw honey or 100 percent organic maple syrup is permitted on a very limited basis.

One-Month Intestinal Restore Cleanse

Shopping List:

> 1 pound pau d'arco bark
> 2 bottles of Integrative Therapeutics Para-Gard (60 veg capsule)
> 1 bottle activated charcoal (I recommend Integrative Therapeutics brand)
> 1 bottle of probiotic capsules or probiotic and/or prebiotic green powder drink such as Green Vibrance
> 1 bottle of L-Glutamine powder (I recommend Thorne brand)
> Optional: Additional loose-leaf herbal teas to add to the pau d'arco medicinal tea elixir: red clover, burdock, sarsaparilla, dandelion, dandelion root, and echinacea.

Day 1 to 14 of Intestinal Restore Cleanse

Morning: Drink 1/2 liter of tea brewed from pau d'arco. Feel free to add other antifungal and immune-boosting herbs as well. Helpful herbs to add in the purification of the blood and the detox process include red clover, burdock, sarsaparilla, dandelion, dandelion root, and echinacea. Take a probiotic capsule or scoop of green drink with breakfast.

Breakfast Ideas: Egg with avocado omelet, whole grain oatmeal with 1 tablespoon coconut oil and chopped walnuts.

Lunch Ideas: Chicken and vegetable soup, lentil soup, split pea soup, mixed greens salad made with dressing containing all natural oils (avocado oil, olive oil, coconut oil).

HOW TO BREW HOMEMADE
MEDICINAL HERBAL TEA ELIXIRS

In a stainless steel pot, boil desired amount of water. As soon as the water starts to boil, add 1 to 3 tablespoons of bark and herbs per cup of water. Boil for 5 minutes, then turn the heat off and allow the herbs to infuse for an additional 5 to 20 minutes to your desired strength. The longer they infuse the more nutrients will be extracted from the herbs. Add lemon or sweeten with stevia or raw organic honey for flavor. Make sure that the tea is brewed strong enough to taste a distinct flavor. If it's not palatable, it's better to drink 2 liters of a weaker brewed tea that is palatable than two glasses of tea brewed too strong leaves you with a headache. A great source of high-quality tinctures, pau d'arco bark, and dried herbs is found at http://www.mountainroseherbs.com.

Afternoon: Drink 1/2 liter of brewed antifungal tea and 1/2 liter of water. Take 2 capsules of Para-Gard after eating and 1 teaspoon of L-Glutamine powder.

Evening: Take 2 capsules of Para-Gard after eating and 2 capsules of activated charcoal. Drink 1/2 liter of brewed antifungal tea or other herbal tea of your choice (mint tea, chamomile, licorice root tea).

Dinner Ideas: Salad topped with grilled chicken and vegetables, or salmon with miso dressing and vegetables.

Sweet-Fix Snacks: Trail mix with carob bits; apple with all-natural, no-sugar nut butter; chopped almonds blended with Medjool dates and 1 teaspoon cacao powder in a food processor.

Day 14 to 30 of Intestinal Restore Cleanse

Morning: Drink 1/4 liter of antifungal tea and 1/4 liter of water. Take a probiotic capsule or green drink with food.

Afternoon: Take 1 capsule of Para-Gard with food and 1 teaspoon L-Glutamine powder.

Evening: Take 1 capsule of Para-Gard with food and 1 capsule of activated charcoal. Drink 1 cup of herbal tea of your choice.

TAKEAWAYS

- Microbes make up over 99 percent of the genetic material in our bodies and have a huge influence on the remaining 1 percent inherited from our parents.

- Our gut flora promotes normal gastrointestinal functions such as nutrient absorption and digestion, provides protection from infection, regulates metabolism, and comprises more than 75 percent of the immune system in the form of the mucosal immune system.
- Antibiotics and other medical interventions, high blood sugar, and a weakened immune system can lead to an overgrowth of *Candida albicans* or other pathogenic microbes in the intestinal tract.
- *Candida* overgrowth can contribute to unstable blood sugar and sugar cravings.
- A small amount of *Candida* is normal and plays a role in microbial balance. However, when this yeast starts to outnumber the level of friendly bacteria and fungi in the blood, it can compromise the entire immune system as the yeast continues to multiply by feeding on blood sugar.

· 4 ·

A Sweet Addiction

[F]ood, instead of being my most direct link with the nurturing earth had become mere merchandise by which I fulfilled my role as a "good" customer.

—Frances Moore Lappé, *Diet for a Small Planet*

Standing in the café, I lift the oven-fresh cookie to my mouth and watch the steam rising in spirals from the surface, warming my face and filling my nostrils with the scent of cinnamon and chocolate. Biting into the sweet goodness in my hand, I feel my face relax and eyes soften. Chocolate oozes out of the sides and melts on my tongue. Somewhere in the depths of my brain, a powerful surge of the neurotransmitter dopamine is being released in my nucleus accumbens—the "pleasure centers." They lock into my dopamine receptors, and I experience a temporary feeling of euphoria. In this moment all my personal problems melt away, and in this brief amnesia, only this soft, gooey, crispy dessert is the object of my desire.

We all should know that sugar is bad for us, so why do we continue to consume massive quantities of fluffy, powdered confections every year? The average American consumes three pounds of added sugar each week—or 3,550 pounds in their lifetime. The biggest culprits, in order of consumption, are soft drinks; candy, cakes, cookies, and pies; fruit juice; dairy-based desserts and milk; and other baked goods. Translated into calories, this comes to about 500 calories of added sugar every day, which is equivalent to ten strips of bacon.[1] Even if you don't drink soda or are well below this U.S. average sugar intake, you still may be consuming much more than you realize and could be suffering from sugar's effects. That's because an "average" amount of sugar consumption in the United States (16 percent of total daily caloric intake) is still double the sugar consumption of the rest of the world (8 percent of total daily caloric intake).[2] When we compare ourselves to countries like China,

51

they put us to shame with only 2 percent of their daily calories attributed to sugar and sweeteners. Our culture's over-the-top sugar consumption is by no means a new phenomenon; these statistics have in fact remained consistent since 1960.

Why can't we seem to help it? Well, on some level we really can't. The last thing anyone needs to be told for the millionth time is to stop eating sugary processed foods. We all *know* sugar is bad for us, yet there's no doubt that humans derive substantial pleasure from eating sugary sweets. What we need is help quitting these foods. I'm not going to beat around the cane bush here—sugar is *extremely* addictive. Eating fifty grams of sugar every day and telling yourself that you won't form an addictive habit is like smoking a pack of cigarettes every day and telling yourself you won't get hooked.

According to brain scans, sugar is as addictive as cocaine and can be harder to cut out of our diet than quitting smoking.[3, 4] In studies, rats preferred sugar water to cocaine up to the point that the effort required for them to attain the sugar water was eight times more than the effort required to attain cocaine. Arguably, we humans also seem to prefer sugar with its low-grade stimulant effect and dopamine release to the intensity of other stimulants like nicotine and recreational drugs. Common sugar withdrawal symptoms—besides the more obvious sugar cravings—include feeling lightheaded, anxious, depressed, irritable, tired, and muscle aches, and headaches. Researchers at Princeton University found that the withdrawal signs from sugar were similar to withdrawal from nicotine, morphine, and other opioids due to the comparable acetylcholine-dopamine imbalance in the brain—two neurotransmitters most affected by chemical dependencies.[5]

The dopamine spike in your brain is not the only reward you get from consuming sugar. Sugar in the form of granulated sugars and fruit juice also cause a literal sugar high from the quick conversion of sucrose into glucose in our bloodstream, as we've discussed. We will go over use of sugar as a stimulant more in chapter 5, "Be Mindful of the Stress-Induced Sweet Tooth." For now, suffice it to say that when used as a stimulant, the high will only last anywhere from one to twenty minutes, depending on how much sugar you ate and your individual tolerance level, and then you're right back where you started—and often more tired, hungry, and cranky than before.

VOTE WITH YOUR WALLET

Processed food companies know all too well how addictive their foods are. This is the reason they are among the most powerful companies in the world.

If we eat sugary foods multiple times a day on a regular basis, a tidal wave of glucose repeatedly floods our system throughout the day. Dopamine is a neurotransmitter that is released every time we do something we find enjoyable. But unlike enjoyable activities that contribute to our health and well-being, like going for a long walk or playing with our children, sugar raises the level of inflammation in the body in addition to precipitating weight gain, blood sugar problems, and a whole host of inflammatory illnesses. It's also incredibly hard to quit, because we can partake of sugar no matter where we are and at any time of the day—in fact, sugar consumption today is often likened to smoking before indoor and workplace smoking laws were enacted. As recently as the early 1990s, smokers could smoke at restaurants, work, bus and train stations, and at home. Everyone could chain-smoke all day long, no matter where they were! California was the first state to enact a statewide smoking ban in enclosed public places, in 1995. Now, smoke-free laws prohibit smoking in most public places, even in many city apartment buildings. Of course, I wouldn't go so far as to say we should outlaw sugar in public places, but could it be that there are places where it simply doesn't make sense to have diverse quantities of sweet confections available? Should we have massive amounts of sugar in schools, hospitals, and pharmacies—after all, these are places that are supposed to support our health and well-being, right?

Choosing what types of foods you buy and where is indeed a political act in a world where processed food giants limit our access to local, fresh, organic, wholesome foods. We can talk all day about how our primitive ancestral brains are hardwired to crave and eat sweet foods, and I'm not arguing against this fact, but that's like saying the reason everybody smoked Marlboro cigarettes in 1950 was because they had no self-control—manipulative marketing techniques swayed them to inhale from a bitter burning roll of paper and that was it, one cigarette and they were hooked for life. Now we know that cigarettes are extremely addictive and harmful, and the rate of smoking continues to go down every day. Why? Because we collectively learned how to *tune out* manipulative tobacco industry marketing tactics and *tune in* to self-care, but only after universal acceptance of the harmful short- and long-term health effects of cigarettes and the addictiveness of nicotine. Today we know for certain that smoking is deadly and addictive, but do we say the same about highly processed, sugary foods?

What does the food industry want? This question doesn't require much brain power. Every company that makes packaged or processed food has the same aim—to get people addicted to their food and eat more and more of their goods. In other words, their goal is simple: to make it easy and enjoyable to overeat. Governed by the laws of capitalism, as people buy more goods, the supply of these products goes down and the price goes up. This is based on the assumption that there is nothing stopping you from buying the products except your bank account. Food companies run into a bit of a hitch compared to other products in the world of supply and demand. A person will not buy more food than they can feasibly consume, no matter how fat their wallet is. This is why large food corporations build giant labs and run thousands of experiments to create market-approved flavors that we can eat in addition to our breakfast, lunch, and dinner, or store on a shelf for five to ten years. The richest and most powerful people in our country are literally putting millions of dollars into research development and marketing to convince people to eat food that is closer to the nutritional value of cardboard than actual food. This is the genius of sweets and snack foods. These foods, conceived in a laboratory, have few if any real nutrients left in them, and this is why they are not satisfying and often leave you feeling hungry, despite containing loads of added sugar or refined flours. Any vitamins or minerals claimed to have been added back in afterward are equivalent to taking one-eighth of a low-grade multivitamin at best.

Food companies spend billions of dollars every year marketing their products to us. It's impossible to conceive that we are *not* affected by this to some degree. In 2013 the food and beverage industry spent a total of $136.53 million on advertising.[6] Why would they spend this much money if it was ineffective at getting people to buy and eat their goods? Even the makeup of a supermarket manipulates us into purchasing all these food-like substances. With half the center aisles devoted to cereals, snacks, soda, and cookies, it leads to an unconscious assumption that the same proportion of our diet should come from those foods. There is in fact an entire supermarket psychology behind the way grocery stores are set up.[7] Supermarkets are designed to get customers to spend as much time as possible within their doors. Having the dairy and meat departments almost always located as far from the entrance as possible forces customers—who invariably will have at least one highly perishable item on their list—to walk through all the middle isles of snacks and packaged foods on their way to the milk, eggs, cheese, yogurt, and meat. The rationale, of course, is the longer you stay in the store, the more stuff you'll see and want to buy. According to brain-scan experiments, after about forty minutes of shopping, most people stop making rational shopping choices and begin shopping based on what they want in that moment. This is when 50 percent of the items we purchase, but never intended to buy, end up in our cart.[8]

SUGAR CHEMISTRY 101

With all the research out there on the addictiveness of sucrose and the physiological processes of blood sugar spikes and release of dopamine and other neurochemicals in our brains, it's not such a leap to assume that other foods can cause a similar effect on our brains, albeit to a slightly lesser degree. When most of us think of the term *sugar*, we imagine the stuff that comes in colorful candy wrappers or in frosting on a cake, not in sandwiches, wraps, and on our dinner plate. If you take a scientific look at sugar, the definition becomes much broader. The names for sugar in microbiology are monosaccharides and disaccharides. Monosaccharide comes from the Greek words *mono* (single) and *sacchar* (sugar) and includes galactose (dairy), glucose (fruits, high-carbohydrate foods), and fructose (fruit). These forms of sugar are the simplest and easiest for the body to assimilate into the bloodstream.

Disaccharides, or double sugars, contain two monosaccharides. Common disaccharides in our diet are sucrose (table sugar, cane sugar), lactose (milk sugar), and maltose (used to make beer). Double sugars split apart easily, which allows glucose to flood our bloodstream quickly. This process is what makes refined sugar, skim milk, and grains like refined wheat flour much worse for our blood sugar, digestion, and microbiome compared to less processed foods like whole-fat milk products such as yogurt, hearty oatmeal, or potatoes. Here's a breakdown of all the double sugars found in our food:

Sucrose = glucose + fructose
Lactose = glucose + galactose
Maltose = glucose + glucose

The more processed and refined the carbohydrate, the faster it breaks down into its corresponding monosaccharides in the body and the bigger the sugar rush. This is why refined and processed grains such as bread and other baked goods can have a dangerous metabolic effect on blood sugar when consumed in high amounts or without sufficient fat, protein, and fiber. However, foods that contain a higher proportion of fiber (whole fruits, potatoes, beans, lentils, whole grains), fat (nuts, cheese, whole cream), or protein (yogurt, legumes, certain whole grains) initiate smaller waves of glucose entering the blood, making it easier for the body to maintain the desired blood sugar balance. Certain complex carbohydrates such as beans and many whole grains (whole oats, buckwheat,[9] millet, and amaranth) have also been shown to feed our beneficial bacteria in addition to helping maintain a balanced blood sugar level by improving insulin sensitivity.[10]

Ever heard of a refined carbohydrate addict? A hundred years ago, the disaccharides in mill-ground flours came with sufficient starch and fiber to offset the effect of a glucose spike. Nowadays, due to the high-tech manufacturing process of flour and other grains, our bread and other baked goods are having a similar effect as table sugar on our bodies—entering our blood so fast it's like a tidal wave hitting calm waters—and causing serious health consequences. Glucose found in refined carbohydrates, like crackers and white bread, has the same glycemic index as white table sugar. This wears down our insulin receptors over time and spikes blood sugar in much the same way as sugar, resulting in similar effects on the dopamine and opioid receptors in the brain. Psychology researchers are now developing therapies for refined food addiction in order to provide helpful therapeutic interventions to treat this very real phenomenon.[11] In the words of researchers exploring food addiction at the Refined Food Addiction Research Foundation (ReFA): "Psychoactive substances disrupt the very emotions that evolved to regulate our behavior. They arouse reward mechanisms artificially, thus stimulating the circuits that are normally fired by events that provide a huge gain; but they provide no gain. They simply create an illusion."[12] In other words, our body thinks we are receiving a lot of nutrition, when in actuality we are only receiving empty calories, a.k.a. sugar.

In refined sugars, milk, and flours, the sugars and carbohydrates are stripped of the fibrous, fatty, or protein-rich portion of the plant such as the husk or shell, or in the case of skim milk, the more nutritious cream, leaving primarily the sugars to be consumed. Skim milk, purported as healthier than whole-fat milk, really should be called *refined milk* and likened to refined flour or refined sugar due to its high sugar content. One glass of skim milk can contain up to thirty grams of sugar! Skim milk has developed a reputation of being more diet-friendly than whole milk because it contains less fat per serving, but it acts a lot like sugar in the body, leading to blood sugar spikes and dips that wear down insulin receptors and result in sugar cravings afterward. In the refining process of skim milk, all the fat—which coincidentally is the part of the milk containing the majority of the vitamins and nutrients found in milk—is stripped out, leaving only lactose and a tiny bit of protein—not enough to offset the lactose content and prevent a blood sugar spike. Fats, the previous culprit in weight gain, have been trumped by sugar. We now know healthy fats actually protect us against weight gain by increasing our satiety after meals through their stimulation of leptin and balancing of blood sugar. Whole, non–refined grains such as wheat berries, brown rice, and quinoa, for example, contain protein, fiber, and other nutrients that prevent this blood sugar spike, and therefore don't have the same addictive or insulin resistant qualities.

Wondering what types of sugars are in your food? It's always important to check the ingredients listed to see what types of "natural sugars," such as fruit sugar from whole fruit or fruit juice, and "refined sugars," such as table sugar, conventional honey, and high-fructose corn syrup are in your food.

SUGAR LEVELS, DOPAMINE,
AND THE RAT STUDY

In 2008 at the annual meeting of the American College of Neuropsycho-pharmacology, a team of researchers from Princeton, led by Professor Bart Hoebel, presented a study demonstrating how rats exhibit three elements of addiction in response to changes in sugar levels in their diets.[13] Dopamine had already been found in numerous other studies to trigger motivation and, with repetition, addiction. They monitored the rats' brains closely and found that dopamine was released in the brain when hungry rats would "binge" on a sugar solution. This "sugar-bingeing" is characterized by neurochemical changes in the brain that mimic those produced by substances of abuse, including nicotine, cocaine, and morphine. The researchers were able to observe a distinct pattern of addictive behavior starting with increased intake, or bingeing, on the sugar solution, followed by signs of withdrawal when they weren't given the same amount of sugar in their diet, then by cravings and relapse. The behavioral pattern captured in their experiments showed long-lasting effects in the brain as well, such as increased inclination to take other drugs of abuse—for example, alcohol.

After a month the rats' brains adapted to the increased dopamine levels by showing fewer dopamine receptors and more opioid receptors. This biological change is a typical response when there is an increased dependence on a substance, such as nicotine, alcohol, cocaine, or other drugs. When the researchers removed the sugar supply, the levels of dopamine in the brains of the rats dropped, and they became anxious, as demonstrated by their chattering teeth and choice to remain in dark tunnels rather than venturing out to play in their playground maze—clear signs of withdrawal.

In a similar study in 2007, researchers at James Cook University in Australia also discovered that cocaine-addicted mice preferred sugar water as a reward over cocaine.[14] Humans are much more intelligent and evolved than mice, of course, but the relationship between sugar consumption, effects on the brain, and the behavior patterns that follow can teach us a lot about the biological aspect of food addiction and even eating disorders. Studies like this demonstrate that there's a euphoria from sugar consumption powerful enough to cause us to reach for sugar more often than we may even realize, despite the negative side effects of disrupted insulin and blood sugar control, overgrowth of pathogenic flora in the gut, increased hunger, addictiveness, withdrawal symptoms, and triggering of inflammatory pathways in the body.

Our nation's sugar habits are more dangerous than previously thought in the scientific community. Even low to moderate sugar and refined carbohydrate consumption has been shown in numerous studies to impair the metabolism of sugar and fat and promote inflammation in healthy subjects.[15, 16, 17] Inflammation has been shown to lead to heart disease, cancer, arthritis, and a host of digestive disorders. Consuming refined sugar is now linked to obesity, hypertension, high blood pressure, diabetes, hypoglycemia, acne, migraines, and many other chronic conditions, especially when coupled with stress.[18] According to a new study presented at the 58th Annual Scientific Meeting of the American Headache Society—an annual meeting that draws 1,000 headache and migraine researchers and treatment specialists from around the world—a common biomarker of inflammation, C-reactive protein, was found to be associated with migraines and cardiovascular and stroke risk in young adults. The study found that participants with migraines had significantly higher than average levels of inflammation than those without migraines.[19]

What is inflammation? Inflammation is not always bad. If you get a cut or a scrape, your body will rev up your immune system to fight off an infection, turning the area red and swollen—that's your inflammatory response at work. But there's a difference between inflammation from an injury and inflammation in your intestinal gut lining. After an injury, eventually the cut will heal and everything will go back to normal. But imagine you keep scraping yourself over and over without any rest time in between to let your body repair. The inflammation will never go down because you're constantly re-injuring yourself. This is what happens when your gut lining is continually irritated. The list of factors that can irritate our microbiome and gut lining is long and includes stress,[20] certain medications, sugar, and other refined high-glycemic foods. Stress alone has been shown to increase intestinal permeability and cause inflammation in the gut and dysregulation of the gut-brain-axis, leading to a long list of disorders in the GI tract.[21] In the case of processed, refined, sugary food habits, the injury may be being repeated three meals a day, or more with snacks, 365 days a year!

AN UNKNOWN TOXIN, FRUCTOSE

The liver, responsible for detoxifying the blood, also plays an important part in the digestion of sugar. As we mentioned earlier, fructose (also found in sucrose or table sugar) is 100 percent digested by the liver. Once fructose makes it to the liver, it is converted to glucose, which is then converted to glycogen and lactate. Even though only a small amount of fructose reaches the bloodstream, it still has an impact on your blood sugar.

Back in the 1990s, refined fructose developed a positive reputation in regard to balancing blood sugar, on the basis that it is digested through the liver. It was theorized that it must be good for blood sugar because it does not cause a high blood sugar spike. More recent research, however, shows that fructose, unlike glucose, does not cause insulin to be released or stimulate the production of leptin, a hormone that sends the signal to our body that we've had enough to eat. The metabolism of fructose by your liver also creates toxins such as uric acid, which drives up blood sugar and can cause gout. Most important, though, is that much of the fructose in the fruit juice and table sugar that you eat is turned into free fatty acids, damaging cholesterol (VLDL) and triglycerides, which get stored as adipose tissue surrounding your organs. Basically, fructose turns directly into fat—and mainly belly fat.[22] Of course, when consumed in the form of a whole fruit, the hit to the liver is much more gradual, and there is a much lower lipogenic effect compared to table sugar. Take a pear versus pear juice, for example. When you drink pear juice, it quickly delivers a lot of fructose to your liver and glucose to your blood. However, when you eat a whole pear, the added fiber and other compounds slow digestion and cause the sugar to be released more gradually, sustaining you for longer until the next meal.

Because of this unique way our body processes fructose, when we consume refined sugars, it has a similar effect to alcohol in that it creates a huge burden on our liver and gets in the way of our body's natural detox process—the way in which the body rids itself of environmental toxins and sheds excess weight. Because of the role our liver plays in processing fructose, it is treated much like other toxins in the way our body protects itself. When our system gets overrun with toxins—due to our detox process being inhibited by continuous intake of sugar, alcohol, and refined foods, among other factors such as chronic stress and medication use—excess toxins will bind to gene signaling within white adipose tissue. Signaling pathways control cell growth and are expressed by genes. The order is thus communicated through signaling proteins to store the excess fructose and other toxins in fat cells to protect our vital organs from exposure.[23] If our liver is already burdened by sugar, microenvironmental exposure to fat-soluble toxins such as chlorine, heavy metals, pesticides, preservatives, food additives, pollutants, plastics, and other common environmental chemicals, which we are exposed to through our modern food and drinking water, has a cumulative effect that puts added stress on the immune system and has a detrimental effect on our supply of beneficial gut bacteria—all of which makes it much more likely we will get sick. Our everyday environment, laden with processed, packaged foods with a high toxic load, is literally creating the ideal breeding ground for pathogenic flora overgrowth and even cancer cell growth. Research shows a clear link between the pH of our body and cancer.[24] Cancer thrives in an acidic environment and cannot survive in a healthy, alkaline human body.[25]

We need our microbiome now more than ever. Our microbiome plays a role of utmost importance in supporting our natural detox process—our most powerful defense against our continuous exposure to toxins that we can't help but come into contact with in our modern world. Of course there are many actions we can take to limit exposures to plastics, chlorine, food additives, pesticides, antibiotics, herbicides and other chemicals which harm our microbiome, but the single most effective thing we can do is bolster the health of our gut microbial environment to support our immune system and liver in excreting any micro-exposures to chemicals we come into contact with on a daily basis. An added benefit is that doing so often results in nearly effortless weight loss. If you're interested in learning more about alkaline foods, search for "Alkaline/Acid Food Charts" online to see which alkaline foods can help restore your body to its desirable pH.

MY SUGAR OVERLOAD

I remember when sneaking into the kitchen late in the night for a sweet snack was a common occurrence in my life. The year after graduating college and moving into an apartment with my boyfriend, I often found myself sneaking off to eat sweets at odd hours of the day and night. Responding to the cravings, I'd open the refrigerator and pull out a slice of leftover chocolate cake, telling myself, *I'm only going to take one bite.* Of course, on some level I knew I was lying to myself, but before I would even have time to process that thought, I had devoured the thick slice of cake.

Sound familiar? Given that you are reading this book, chances are you have found yourself in a similar predicament before as well. Maybe like me, eating sugar and processed carbs allows you a momentary break or distraction from your to-do list. Temporarily at least, it gives you a break from your anxieties as you drift into the dopamine-derived sensation of eating a delicious sweet. Not long after, though, if you're like me, you likely feel awful—guilty, perhaps bloated, devoid of energy, and soon, very hungry again from the sudden blood sugar drop, which may lead you to seek more sugar than before. And so the cycle continues.

Once I found out that sugar was tipping the scales in my intestinal lining to produce inflammation and feed *Candida albicans*, causing many of my mysterious symptoms, I consulted with a holistic doctor who told me to stop eating all refined flour, fruit juice, and sugar to stop the overgrowth of candidiasis that had colonized my gut so completely it had spread from my intestines into my bloodstream. The best way to kill off an army? Starve it to death. It was then that I made the resolution to cut sugary foods out of my diet for three months.

For me the task of learning which foods contained high-glycemic ingredients and were harming my microbiome was daunting. I decided to start with the most obvious suspect—refined table sugar. The most current research I found on sugar showed added sugar hiding in 74 percent[26] of packaged foods we buy in the grocery store, including many foods promoted as "healthy." For example, many leading brands of yogurt contain up to twenty-nine grams of sugar per serving, with refined sugar listed in the first three ingredients on the food label. That's more refined sugar than we should be consuming in an entire day! I discovered that it was difficult to find a single packaged snack item on the shelves of my local grocery store that didn't contain loads of sugar or refined flour.

I was not very practiced at ignoring sugar's call at the time. In fact, you could say I had refined the art of seeking out and finding my favorite sugary foods. Whether I was consciously seeking it, or desiring it on a subconscious level, it seemed no matter where I was, sugar and refined wheat products were laid out in front of me, free for the taking. Sugar permeated my landscape and my every move, oozing out of the breakroom at work in the form of endless snacks, doughnuts, and coffee creamers. It waited for me at the frozen yogurt place on the corner as I walked down the street to buy a healthy lunch. It taunted me from the endless rows of chocolate candy, and even right at the checkout counter while I waited in line at the pharmacy, of all places—a place I buy medicines when sick! I even found it hiding in my supposedly "healthy" snacks, including granola bars, cereals, breads, yogurts, ketchup, and other foods.

CAN WE EAT SUGAR WITHOUT FORMING AN ADDICTIVE HABIT?

As is the case with smoking, sugar consumption on a regular basis, such as multiple times a day, eventually leads the brain to compensate for the consistent blood sugar high by reducing the number of dopamine receptors. With a reduction in dopamine receptors, the high from increased dopamine starts to lose its effect unless we flood it with even more sugar, more frequently, leading to a classic addictive cycle. Just like with any drug, if we are engaged in this type of addictive behavior with sugary foods on a daily basis, small doses of natural dopamine slowly start to have less of an impact on the brain's reward center. Soon, natural surges of dopamine, such as those that come from a hot shower, the relief at the end of a long workday, or a kiss from a loved one, are a little less stimulating than they used to be. Then we start to seek stronger and stronger sensations of stimulation and relaxation, such as more intense sweet stuff, and we look for it more often.

The only way to eat sugar without forming a bad habit is to stop eating it long enough for your brain to go through withdrawal from the sugar-induced dopamine it has come to rely on. This often produces symptoms such as muscle aches, headaches, and feeling lightheaded, anxious, depressed, irritable, and fatigued. The time frame for these symptoms varies depending on the individual but typically doesn't last longer than two to five days. Then, after a period of one to three months, spent rebuilding healthy gut flora and balancing blood sugar, when small amounts of sugar—and better yet, healthy, low-glycemic alternatives such as organic coconut sugar or lucuma fruit powder—are allowed back in the diet on a sporadic basis, rather than daily, you can enjoy the effects of sugar without allowing the brain to form a habit where dependence increases over time. The amount of time it takes to break a dependence on sugar can be different for everyone, but if it's your first time cutting out refined sugar in your diet for an extended period of time, it can take two to four weeks for most people to detox from sugar's biological effects, and up to six months if you suffer from severe candida. When you do reintroduce sugar, which you can do as long as it's done mindfully, the key is to limit it to places you do not frequent on a regular basis—for example, special occasions such as holidays, weddings, birthdays, and vacations. Avoid eating sugar all alone at your desk or on your couch at home! That will just lead you right back into an addictive cycle, and you'll have to start all over.

TAKEAWAYS

- Sugar lights up the same parts of the brain as cocaine, is largely stored as fat, and is extremely addictive.
- Comfort eating and refined food addiction is being explored as a disorder in order to provide therapeutic interventions to dealing with addiction to foods.
- Sugar and high-glycemic foods increase inflammation in the body and have been linked to obesity, hypertension, high blood pressure, diabetes, hypoglycemia, acne, migraines, and many other chronic conditions.
- Sugar intake puts stress on the liver, which impedes the body's natural detoxification process, thus increasing acidity, weight gain, inflammation, and chronic disease.
- Cutting out refined sugars for a period of time allows your body a reset. After a period of time, small amounts of sugar can be reintroduced mindfully.

Be Mindful of Your Stress-Induced Sweet Tooth

Until you make the unconscious conscious, it will direct your life and you will call it fate.

—Carl Jung

$\mathscr{R}$esearchers at the University of California–Davis found that 80 percent of people report eating more sweets when they are under stress.[1] If you've also noticed a tendency to crave sugar and make poorer choices in your diet at the end of a long, busy day, you're not alone. We live in a world that demands we be at our peak performance all day at work and then be attentive and present with our partner and children when we are home, running errands, cleaning up, cooking dinner, or doing a number of other things. This expectation is nearly impossible to satisfy. It's easy to reach for stimulants during a busy day without even thinking about it, simply to keep going when our body is about to give out.

THE CORTISOL TRIP

After cutting out sugar for a month, I was feeling more energetic, losing weight, noticing clearer skin, and had a stronger immune system—as evidenced by less frequent illnesses. Yet my motivation to stay away from sugar would often weaken when my stress peaked. As I continued to look deeper, I started to piece together that the main culprit was a constant anxious back chatter in my mind triggering a physiological stress response. Our stress response causes our bodies to think we need cortisol and adrenaline, two hormones created and secreted by our adrenal glands to help us deal with a stressful situation. Add to that my irregular sleep patterns—poor-quality sleep is also a common cause of elevated cortisol and adrenaline—and I had a big problem. Even though my anxiety continued to dwindle as I took steps to heal my gut, my body's stress response was still stuck in overdrive, and I didn't know how to stop it!

As mentioned in chapter 3, there is a whole nervous system that exists entirely in our gut, called the enteric nervous system (ENS). Also called the intrinsic nervous system, our ENS is a vast network of neurons (500 million neurons) spread throughout two layers of gut tissue in our large and small intestines. The ENS is one of three subdivisions of the autonomic nervous system. Our autonomic nervous system acts mostly unconsciously, regulating functions such as heart rate, digestion, respiratory rate, and sexual arousal by sending neurotransmitters to our organs. The other two divisions of the autonomic nervous system are much more widely known due to their influence on "fight or flight" mode, as directed by the sympathetic nervous system, or relax and digest mode, as directed by our parasympathetic nervous system. Our gut communicates with our central nervous system (brain and spinal cord) through sympathetic and parasympathetic nerve fibers to provide sensory information, and our brain communicates back affecting digestion and other gastrointestinal function. There are literally hundreds of millions of neurons communicating between our gut and our brain within this network. In one giant feedback loop messaging is firing in both directions. Ninety percent of the signals that pass through the vagus nerve—the primary mode of communication between our body and our brain—come from the enteric nervous system.[2] Our mental strain, worry, and fear—sent as messages from our brain to our gut—can weaken our digestive system and lead to microbial imbalance and a whole host of other health issues. Our stress response decreases nutrient absorption, lowers oxygen levels, and reduces blood flow to the gut, which slows metabolism and decreases enzymatic activity and output in the gut—as much as 200 times less activity. This contributes further to the poor nutrient absorption of our food.[3] Whether a result of cortisol levels running too high on a consistent basis, impaired gastrointestinal function, or both, chronic stress will lead to imbalanced microbial biodiversity and nutrient deficiencies if not addressed.[4] Our psychological stress further increases the permeability of the gut, in a similar way that certain food products like refined wheat and sugar do. When our intestinal wall is weakened, bacteria and bacterial antigens can cross the epithelial intestinal wall, triggering a pro-inflammatory mucosal immune response.[5] Partially digested food particles can also cross this wall, triggering an autoimmune response to those foods.

Stress also disrupts our blood sugar, independent of our diet. How does it do that? When we are under stress, our body releases excess cortisol, which causes the liver to release glucose. This heightened stress can cause a severe blood sugar spike, as if we just ate a load of sugary foods, even if we didn't! A state of fear often required our ancestors to either run or fight for their lives, and the extra shot of glucose served as fuel. Those who received the biggest glucose spike when in danger were more likely to survive. By evolutionary logic then, as the offspring of those survivors, we have the most effective glucose spike. Even if we don't need this extra glucose spike in to-day's modern world, as a species we have evolved to respond this way. This activates a sugar pendulum in much the same way sugary foods do. Soon our pancreas gets the signal that our blood sugar is too high and produces insulin to activate our cells to take in glucose. When insulin levels rise, our cells take in the excess glucose, causing our blood sugar to plummet, result-ing in stress-induced sweet cravings, which is the body's way of screaming, *Give me more glucose!* This yo-yo of blood sugar inconsistency, triggered by cortisol and insulin, can quickly start to wear out our body's response to insulin. The resulting cycle creates a metabolic-brain negative feedback pathway affected by sugar and, for many stressed-out individuals, a higher incidence of sugar addiction and weight gain, according to findings at the University of California–Davis. In another study published in the *Journal of Clinical Endocrinology and Metabolism*, cortisol levels were tested via the hair samples of 283 older men and women over a three-month period, and it was found that the participants with higher levels of cortisol had three times the risk for cardiovascular disease and diabetes.[6]

When we are dealing with long-term stress, our body is constantly—for months or even years—in what should only be a short-term "fight or flight mode." Back in our hunter-gatherer days, this state was an appropriate re-sponse when running away from a tiger, foraging for food for our starving family, or killing a predator. Our body needed adrenaline to perform these sorts of physical and heroic feats. These days when we encounter a stressful situation, like our stocks plummeting, our manager calling us in for a meet-ing, or the hairdresser going scissors crazy, it doesn't usually require us to react physically like our ancestors did. The problem is, even though we can reason with ourselves logically that we are not going to die and our hair will grow back, the stress response that is triggered from the social shame we expect to experience is the same as if there was a real threat to our lives. In fact, back in our prehistoric days, social shaming and the threat of abandonment from our tribe *was* equivalent to death, since we likely could not have survived in the wild on our own. Over the millennia, as living conditions have improved and the population has grown, our basic hardwiring hasn't changed. The threat of social shame still feels just as terrifying, even though we no longer rely on societal approval for basic survival.

If the body is secreting high levels of the hormones cortisol and adrenaline on a consistent basis, it is forced to build more of these hormones with the resources available in its internal storage facilities. B vitamins, minerals like magnesium, and other vitamins are stored specifically to build more of these hormones to revive us in times of stress. That's why in the first couple of days after encountering a new stressor, like having a baby, for example, we may not feel stressed despite the loss of sleep, lack of self-care, and guessing games we play with a new infant to figure out what it needs. Vitamins and minerals are released from their stores to make cortisol, replenish us, and manage our stress. But as time goes on and the sleep deprivation continues, or the stressful situation continues, the physiological mechanisms our body has in place to combat the situation begin to break down. Our stored resources are only finite.

We rely on our gut microbes to break down all fruits, vegetables, and other fiber-filled foods into their corresponding nutrients to replenish these stores. If our adrenal glands are using these resources faster than our gut can replenish them, we have a problem. Vitamins D, B5, B6, B12, and C are the core building blocks required to construct the cortisol hormone, which is essential in the function of our adrenal glands. B12, for example, is vital for managing energy levels, forming blood cells, and building the proteins that make up key hormones. Even a short-term deficiency of B12 can lead to decreased progesterone levels and cause hormone imbalance. Meat, eggs, yogurt, and high-protein foods are good sources of B vitamins. Vitamin C helps the body rebuild cell tissues, reduce cellular DNA damage caused by free radicals, and reduce inflammation. Sufficient vitamin D is essential for a healthy functioning endocrine system—the system of glands that produce all the hormones regulating metabolism, tissue function, sexual function, reproduction, sleep, and mood, and more. Vitamin D actually works as a hormone because the body makes it after exposure to the sun; only about 10 percent of vitamin D comes from food or supplements. Unfortunately, today vitamin D deficiency is actually viewed as a pandemic due in part to lack of sun exposure. A lack of fresh seafood naturally containing vitamin D, such as ocean-caught salmon, mackerel, herring, and cod liver oil, compounds the vitamin D deficiency challenge. Very few foods naturally contain vitamin D. Foods that are fortified with vitamin D are inadequate to meet even a child's daily needs. Farmed seafood is much lower in vitamin D, most likely due to the poor diet that farmed fish are given, comprising corn and other grains.[7] Unfortunately, it's very difficult to get enough B12 and D on a strict vegetarian diet, and taking a high-quality B12 and D supplement is a must. High-quality nutritional yeast, like Bragg Nutritional Yeast Seasoning, also contains lots of B vitamins for those avoiding animal products, along with a potent D3 supplement.

Whether from a state of chronic stress or a diet deficient in these nutrients, we may begin to use up all the raw materials used to build cortisol and start to experience the symptoms associated with low levels of these nutrients and stage one adrenal fatigue—sugar cravings, afternoon slump, exercise aversion compensated by snacking, napping, overall reduced physical activity, poor immune system, weak digestion, difficulty concentrating, low-mid back pain, and headaches. If chronic stress continues, adrenal fatigue can then enter into stage two and manifest itself in insomnia, cravings for salty foods, heart palpitations, depression, panic attacks, menstrual irregularity, dizziness, and weight loss. In other words, the symptoms we often associate with stress are actually signs of continuously high cortisol levels leading to *adrenal gland* fatigue and nutrient deficiencies due to poor absorption of nutrients in our gut microbiome.[8] Our adrenals are literally exhausted of all their resources. Pernicious anemia, for example, which is characterized by a B12 deficiency, is associated with chronic fatigue, irritability and frustration, sudden mood swings, impatience, and the desire for isolation.[9, 10] The body is basically shutting down to protect itself from burning out. There is really no way to overestimate both the vital roles that all these vitamins and minerals play in our physical and mental health and how the state of our gut microbiome and enteric nervous system directs how effectively we digest and absorb these nutrients from our diet. This is why, in times of chronic stress, our body requires both mental rest and flora-friendly foods to revive. Research on mindfulness and meditation show that these practices boost immune system function and improve overall health.[11, 12] When compared to relaxation training, meditation training produced autonomic nervous system regulation with significantly less effort, more relaxation of the body, and a longer-lasting calm state of mind afterward.[13]

Our experienced and perceived stress has a direct effect on our microbiome's health, but luckily there's a feedback loop going both ways. The microbiota in our gut also communicates directly with our brain, playing a huge role in regulating our central nervous system. One way your gut flora communicates with your brain and central nervous system is through neurotransmitter production. A number of neurotransmitters, or chemical messengers, are produced by the microbiota in the gut, including dopamine, serotonin, and GABA. This is how the specific assemblage of different species of bacteria in the enteric nervous system influences the development or prevention of autism, anxiety, depression, and other disorders.[14, 15] GABA is the main neurotransmitter produced and utilized by our central nervous system to help us feel a sense of relaxation, calm, and safety. A reduction in GABA production has been implicated in the development of anxiety and depression. Conversely, intake of *lactobacillus*, a common probiotic found in yogurt and other fermented dairy products, has been shown in studies with mice to reduce stress-induced cortisol activity, anxiety, and depression.[16] In a randomized clinical trial in France, human volunteers experienced a reduction in their stress-induced gastrointestinal discomfort in addition to decreased cortisol levels simply by taking a probiotic.[17] Bolstering our microbiome by altering the variety and composition of bacteria in our gut flora may be the underlying problem that needs to be addressed to reduce common symptoms of stress like anxiety, depression, a weakened immune system, and autoimmune disease. It may not be too long before doctors and psychologists alike could be prescribing different microbial cocktails, depending on the illness.[18]

Without a doubt, consuming prebiotic and probiotic foods that contain vital nutrients supports our body in building a diverse microflora to digest and utilize these nutrients efficiently.

To bring permanent change to the distribution of the trillions of bacteria and other flora in our gut, a diverse array of probiotics are vitally important, but alone these little warriors are not enough. Prebiotic supplements and foods are also needed. Leafy greens, algae, sauerkraut, and virtually every other vegetable on the planet play this important role of feeding the good bacteria in the gut. Leafy greens like kale, spinach, and powdered plant-based superfood green drinks like Green Vibrance contain the vital nutrients we need to feed our microflora. When prebiotics are made available to the beneficial flora in our intestines, these flora flourish. Researchers at the Department of Psychiatry at the University of Oxford gave forty-five healthy volunteers a prebiotic supplement and compared them with a placebo group. The researchers found that prebiotics alone significantly decreased high cortisol levels, typically caused by work stressors and often seen in individuals with chronic depression (salivary cortisol reactivity).[19] This study also saw improved attentional bias when volunteers were shown various positive and negative stimuli. Participants literally developed a more positive outlook on life as a result of taking prebiotics. What's more, this study found prebiotics to be as effective as taking SSRI antidepressants like citalopram (Prozac) and benzodiazepines like Valium, often prescribed for anxiety and sleep disturbances, without the negative side effects that come with a pharmacological intervention. Cooking homemade foods with fresh vegetables and making fermented foods may sound daunting at first, but when compared with the costs and side effects of psychotherapy and drugs, it may not seem such a bad trade-off. Why not just buy some cabbage and other leafy green vegetables from a local organic farm at the farmer's market, chock-full of healthy microbes and prebiotic food for your gut, and make yourself some sauerkraut, your own healing homemade cocktail for your gut?

THIS IS LIFE, ON THE GO

A consistently on-the-go, no-rest lifestyle is not compatible with a healthy, happy life and sits in direct opposition to a life of fulfillment and well-being. Developing a new set of microbes that crave flora-friendly foods also requires a slower lifestyle, as our digestive system needs time and rest both during and after meals to properly digest and absorb nutrients. Our capitalist economy's work ethic has us on a nonstop treadmill to increase productivity, all without a moment of stillness or quiet to listen to what our body or heart or *gut* is trying to tell us. When we're caught on this treadmill, we're likely not taking the time to care for our body, such as taking a thirty-minute break from a busy workday to relax and allow our microbes to do their job. Let's stop and think about what we're doing when we blame our stress on our health problems, relationships, work problems, and every other difficult thing in our lives? We're creating this huge beast, encompassing everything from debt, angry bosses, upset children, long commutes, finances, or countless other overwhelming situations in our lives and lumping it all together—effectively stuffing it into a bag we carry over our shoulder all day long, forever enslaving ourselves to this thing called "stress." Why do we do this to ourselves? What I've found from working with many people who share this same experience and whose health is suffering is that, more often than not, we don't *want* to stop. We create our busy lives as a coping mechanism to avoid confronting difficult feelings—fear, sadness, anger, frustration, jealousy. We all do this. We use other distractions too, including food, sweets, television, even exercise, all to avoid facing painful emotions.

At a previous job where I wasn't happy, I developed the habit of eating processed snacks throughout the day. I would grab handful after handful of sweetened popcorn or chocolate chip trail mix and "stuff" it into my mouth. In so doing, I was literally "stuffing" down my dislike of my job, my fear of my boss, all the mistreatment I had endured from her, and all the shame and feelings of worthlessness that accompanied this treatment. At one point, while I was stuffing a handful of chocolate chips in my mouth, I actually had the thought, "I am eating my stress," and then I chewed while thinking about it, gulped, and went back to work. Why? I didn't want to feel it—plain and simple. Eating your feelings sometimes works, in the short term. However, by not taking the time to process these thoughts and emotions and sit with them in mindfulness, I lost sight of the fact that these were merely temporary, situational stressors that I could confront and change in my life. Once I was able to incorporate habits of mindfulness at work, I was able to face my fears, stand up for myself, express my feelings, and take steps toward pursuing a different job that was better suited to meet my needs.

All too often we swat our uncomfortable feelings away, much like an annoying fly buzzing at our ear, yet if we take a moment to listen to that buzzing, we may learn a lot about ourselves and the people around us. The ironic truth is that the more we try to ignore or avoid difficult feelings that trigger us strongly, the more they seep beneath the surface of our awareness and start to become unconscious drivers of our perspectives, reactions, and choices. These difficult feelings become like an undercurrent pulling us along throughout our day, creating our beliefs and setting expectations that shape our everyday experiences. Even if we choose only to see the calm surface of the water—ignoring the tumultuous waves underneath—these feelings are still driving the direction of the current, whether we like it or not.

We can make the choice to move these feelings out of our unconscious and into the light of our awareness every day. Oftentimes it's only in a really difficult situation, in a moment of almost forced surrender, that we do this. Yet our conscious acknowledgment of our innermost feelings doesn't have to—and shouldn't—be this infrequent. If we keep swatting, eventually these little messenger flies will give up and drop out of our awareness. Then months, years, and even decades can go by before we realize it's time to address and listen to those feelings we buried long ago. If years do go by, the buildup may start to feel beyond our control, like we have no power to address this deep, underwater force. However, we do! We don't need to wait until we've reached "rock bottom," so to speak. We can take time each day to give our gut and our heart our ear and our compassion through mindfulness practices like meditation. Welcoming all our emotions, from ecstatic pleasure to unbearable shame, can give our lives new depth of meaning and purpose, again ironically bringing us to a whole new, unimaginable level of contentment. That's because when we cut ourselves off from the difficult emotions, we end up cutting ourselves off from all the good ones, too.

Unfortunately, our feelings don't work in the way we'd like them to. We can't just switch off anger and frustration, leaving only love and ecstasy; whatever feelings we may have, they all come together in one package. In fact, the very emotions that we are trying so hard *not* to feel may be the path to a new perspective or realization that unlocks the door to a new sense of freedom, or to an opening of our hearts to a deeper understanding. This recognition is what creates the much sought-after feeling of connection with ourselves and those around us—*our deepest, one true craving*. The more we acknowledge our fears, the more we will start to hear our deepest desires crying beneath for what we truly yearn for in life. Our most painful feelings can in fact be the key that unlocks these deep desires and callings.

MINDFULNESS TO THE RESCUE

Meditation and mindfulness have gathered a lot of support in recent years as a proven way to reduce stress, anxiety, and depressive symptoms, as well as make CEOs more productive and children play nice. No longer confined to monasteries and Buddhist temples, meditation is being practiced in every major city, in organized classes in schools, at work, at the doctor's office, and in one's own living room. These practices are being integrated into our culture for good reason. Meditation can help us release our chattering mind and drop back into our physical body, tune in to the state of our enteric nervous system, and make decisions from a grounded space of relaxed safety.

Over the last decade, Mindfulness-Based Stress Reduction (MBSR) programs have been found successful in improving anxiety, depression, substance abuse, eating disorders, sleep, and chronic pain, to name a few.[20, 21] The American Heart Association has endorsed meditation and mindfulness as key to lowering the body's stress response. Numerous studies have found mindfulness practices as effective as blood pressure–lowering medication.[22] Several studies, including a recent study published in the *American Journal of Hypertension*, found that after a brief training patients learned how to relax more efficiently, which resulted in significantly lower blood pressure.[23]

Mindfulness has been defined by clinical psychologists as an intentional, heartfelt, nonjudgmental awareness of experiences in the present moment. In other words, mindfulness is a way to reconnect intentionally with our innermost feelings and develop an awareness of our underlying fears and emotions that might be causing us stress. Mindfulness-based stress reduction techniques have been shown to increase well-being and reduce psychiatric and stress–related symptoms by teaching patience, acceptance, and release to help diminish pain sensations and pain-related thoughts.[24, 25]

When we feel worn out, drained, anxious, and fatigued, how often do we still have the energy to cook healthy meals or feel inspiration in any area of our lives? It is not just a state of body or mind, but a state of being that we are addressing. If there is one thing we can learn from our recent findings on the gut biome and our nervous system, it's that there is no separation between the body and the mind. It is one system that needs attention to several components to flourish, much like a flower needs sunshine, soil, and water. Starting with the mind might be the key for you, whereas starting with tending to one's physical health first might work better for someone else. For me personally, and for many of the people I've coached over the years, continually clearing the mind through mindful practices like meditation and yoga helps create a mind-set primed for clarifying goals, coupled with the motivation to create the life we imagine for ourselves. If we all strive to create a state of being that gives us the energy to take on new challenges and feel not only pain-free but comfortable in our bodies too, why do so few of us achieve this?

Just like an irrepressible puppy, our mind will go running after every little thought that catches its attention for even an instant. A dog might jump and chase a squirrel for miles, and to what end? When we tend to the physical sensations in our bodies and intentionally release and relax areas of resistance through mindfulness practices like hatha yoga and meditation, we are training the mind to listen to what our heart and body need, by allowing ourselves to let go, relax, and calm down. The Buddha had a great metaphor that he would use in many of his speeches: "Our mind is like a wild horse. When you train a wild horse, you tie a rope to a post and lead the horse in circles until it has been tamed. When the horse is tamed you can put it to work. If you ask it to ride you from here to there, it does so. If you ask it to plow a field, it does so. In the same way, when we tame our mind, we can put it to work for our own happiness."

Our only alternative to a trained mind is a lifelong chase after one self-critical, distracting, worrisome, reactive thought to the next. This state of being is a tremendous waste of our precious finite energy, which in any given moment could be spent doing much greater, more magnificent things. We are all capable of feeling authentically engaged in our lives with the people, situations, and tasks around us. Taking a second to check in with our true emotions and feelings before acting is a step in the right direction. Taking the time to plan and prepare a healthy lunch so we don't have food guilt when lunchtime rolls around is preferable to opting for the quick, easy meal down the block. We all know this truth already—that taking the easy road out isn't always the best way to solve a problem. The issue is how to tame the mind. How do we start to rein in the spiral of our thoughts? Progress starts with a commitment to ourselves, in every moment, to switch gears.

Perhaps you'll find it most effective to meditate or do yoga or another mindful activity first thing in the morning, so you can carry that mindful state with you while preparing breakfast, packing lunches, or planning what you're going to cook for dinner that night. Once you start to bring this commitment to every area of your life, before you know it you will become more confident not only in your food choices and self-care, but also in your relationships, your family life, and your work.

A regular meditation practice of just twenty minutes a day has been shown to be as effective as therapy, exercise, or medication for anxiety, depression, quality of sleep, immune functioning, attention, memory, managing emotions, chronic pain, and any stress-related illness. Just like any exercise, meditative practice takes time to see results. After three weeks of regular practice, you will start to see these benefits. Visit my website at www.heatherannewise.com to choose from a number of guided meditations recorded by myself and my husband, former Buddhist monk and mindfulness professional, William Jackson, PhD.

Be prepared for your mind to put up a fight. It may not like you saying *no* so often to certain strains of thought that no longer serve you. Your mind also may not take too kindly to you telling it to let go of all the little distractions that have kept it busy for so many years—judgment, gossip, problem solving, and whatever else your mind may cling to. These habits of overthinking are taking up finite space, time, and energy you need to create the life you want. After all, our *thoughts* do eventually become *things* in our lives, whether or not we intend for them to. When attempting to create new mind-sets and beliefs about our life and our health, meditation and mindfulness will make space in our mind and body to integrate these changes fully into our lives. The little "trips" that the mind goes on may have served to entertain us and keep our mind occupied in the past, but now that we have the tools to become more mindful of our thoughts and feelings, we can create positive change in our lives when we let go of these energy-draining thought processes.

Even today, after eight years of having my own meditation practice, I still try to convince myself there are more productive things I can be doing with my mind rather than running through a ten-minute warm-up meditation drill. Much like learning how to play the piano or any instrument, meditation can sometimes feel like playing your daily scales before diving into the piece you want to perform well, or like jogging slow laps prior to running a race or warming up prior to breaking into your favorite dance moves. In the beginning of my meditation my mind often screams, *Get up! Please do something, anything else but focus on a single word like "surrender" or watching the breath go "ah-haaa."* This is so BORING! I often have this fight with my mind when I sit to meditate or do yoga after a busy day of my mind working overtime. Eventually, though, after meditating for five to fifteen minutes, my mind usually gives up the fight and calms down, surrendering to the feelings and emotions underneath my stress. This is where the true healing begins. My body slowly starts to relax, inch by inch, letting go of all the weight my mental strain is putting on it. There is a physical relief in my body and stomach, of my mind finally letting go so I can start to tune in to the state I am in. The outcome is a renewed connection to my inner microbial beings—and a fresh outlook on life. When I make my food and snack choices from this place, after taking a moment of sitting in mindfulness, I am much more apt to choose foods that care for my body and my healthy microbes, rather than harm them.

Meditation and mindful journaling continue to help me develop awareness around all my most common actions and mind-sets and how they affect my digestion, my body, and ultimately my state of health. I invite you to start to incorporate meditation into your busy week. If you are new to meditation, you can begin with meditating just five to ten minutes, three times a week. If you are already a meditation practitioner, challenge yourself to sit for longer and longer periods each week. Bring your awareness to a focal point such as your breath or a mantra that brings you into a state of peace. Maybe it's the image of your child sleeping, or a mantra like "connect" or "release" or "I am whole." You can even use imagery such as light streaming in or the gentle flow of water in a stream. Whatever works to help you find your focus. As you sit, keep bringing your attention back to this focal point. Watch your mind as it wanders to other things you've been worrying about all day, and gently remind it to come back to your mantra or breathing each time it veers away. The more you do this, the more awareness you will develop around the state of your body and how it affects all areas of your life.

If a strong feeling comes up during meditation in the midst of bringing your attention back to your breath, don't push it away. Rather, allow yourself to be curious and sit with it. My meditation space is sometimes the only place I feel safe enough to fully feel a strong emotion that is scary to face. In this way my practice not only gives me some immediate relief from daily stressors, but also helps me process strong feelings that are lurking beneath the surface and unconsciously affecting my life. This practice allows me to peel back the layers of chatter and thoughts to reach the core of a triggering emotional memory or feeling. When I allow myself to sit with an uncomfortable feeling that may arise during my practice, my perception of the feeling or situation changes. Instead of a black-and-white issue or a two-dimensional problem, I start to see a more three-dimensional perspective of a feeling or situation and new solutions to problems. No longer do I see just right or wrong, but rather how a situation came about, how it is progressing, and how it may be solved or passed on its own. In a way, I begin to appreciate the subtle complexity of my experience, which in reality is more like a Rubik's Cube of sides and colors to my feelings that I never saw before.

To give a concrete example, the other day I spoke bluntly about my pregnancy and how rather than always adhering to the warnings about avoiding processed meats and seafoods, I listened to my body and ate whatever my body craved to provide all the nutrients my body was asking for during the course of my pregnancy. After sharing, I was surprised to realize I actually felt isolated from those around me, rather than closer. I thought to myself, *Did I just say something wrong?* It wasn't until later in meditation when I revisited this topic, I realized I was stuck in a subtle mental dichotomy of wondering if it was wrong of me to eat the way I did during my pregnancy.

Alternatively, was it right of me to listen to my body and my instincts, being mindful of the quality of food I was eating and trusting that I would never put myself or my baby at risk? This judgment was rooted mainly in the fear that my choice to take a different path, rather than adhere to strict eating protocols during pregnancy, wouldn't be *accepted* by others. In deciding to share my experience of listening to my body and instincts and doing something slightly different than the "norm," I was also sharing that I had done something taboo, and this was scary! When I spoke, my audience could probably sense that I felt separate, and perhaps they didn't know what to say. At first, when I thought about the situation, I could only see one color. Later, when I sat in meditation I saw all the related feelings and how they fit together, causing me to feel the way I did. Only with this clarity was I finally able to break free from a lingering fear in the periphery of my mind that the group I chose to share with were judging or isolating me. Instead of being stuck in that place of unprocessed worry, I was able to laugh at myself a little, releasing any mental worry that had been following me, and my confidence and trust in my gut were restored.

A NEW RESPONSE TO STRESS AND SUGAR CRAVINGS

As a mother of a high-energy toddler, I often crave sugar when I am worn out, especially in the afternoon or evening after work. Eating refined sugar and grains causes our blood sugar to rise up to ten times faster than any food found in nature. This increase in blood sugar levels acts as a stimulant to your brain and body, giving a short boost of energy and improved cognition. After all, glucose is your brain's fuel too.

In the early months after my daughter was born, the long nights spent nursing every few hours seemed endless. I often turned to stimulants like caffeine and chocolate to stay alert during the day and keep a watchful eye on my child in my sleep-deprived state. Not to mention I was starving all the time during those days of nursing a growing baby. Eating something sweet would temporarily curb my appetite and give me a boost of energy. Yet the kick of my high-glycemic snack would only last for five to fifteen minutes, and afterward I would find myself tired, cranky, and even more ravenously hungry! This led me to, yet again, guiltily grab even more nutrient-deficient, high-carbohydrate foods, and the cycle continued.

This web of fatigue and increasing sugar cravings frustrated me, and wasn't helping me lose the extra weight I'd put on during my pregnancy. One day I started an experiment. After a long day of feeding, entertaining, and cleaning up after my toddler, only to find her in the next room making yet another mess, I was hit with a feeling of fatigue and frustration. Almost immediately, my sweet craving hit *hard*. In that moment, I decided to surrender to that sense of frustration that wanted to be heard and made a conscious decision to tune in to my gut and listen to what it had to say. Instead of reaching for sweets, as I'd gotten in the habit of doing, I intentionally left the mess for twenty minutes and lay down on the couch next to where my daughter was playing to take a rest. While lying there, I started observing my natural breath and quickly noticed, with slight shock, how short and constricted my breathing was. It almost felt as if there was a belt tied tightly around my chest—I couldn't take a single long or relaxed breath. At first, having this realization in the midst of my attempt at a meditative state made me tense up even more, but I refocused on the physical sensations in my body and intentionally brought my awareness to my breath, imagining my chest relaxing and opening, and trusting that my body's state was exactly where it needed to be in that moment. I watched as the belt-like tension slowly started to release and subside. Lying there watching my breath, I consciously released my to-do list and worries, and my breathing began to change. I noticed my breath lengthen and my diaphragm relax. As soon as my breathing was flowing in this more relaxed state, my cravings for sugar disappeared!

If you find that your body is stuck in fight-or-flight mode, it means your sympathetic nervous system is running the show, which will impact your digestion, absorption, and assimilation of nutrients and may trigger sweet craving. For someone new to mindfulness activities, it takes about ten to twenty minutes of mindful meditation or yoga to trigger the parasympathetic nervous system to switch into a relaxation response.[26] Of course, the more you practice mindfulness, the more quickly and effectively the relaxation response can be triggered by simple actions such as bringing attention to physical sensations in the body or to the breath.

Next time you find yourself in a state of overwhelm and have the urge to reach for a sweet stimulant to keep going, I challenge you to make the conscious choice in the moment not to keep going full speed, but to give yourself a five-minute break to listen to what your body is really craving. Find a private, quiet place and take a moment to stop doing whatever you are doing and simply observe. On the surface it may seem like your body is craving a stimulant because your body is stuck with its sympathetic nervous system running on high. On a deeper level, however, maybe your body actually wants to stop for five to ten minutes to reset, switching back to the parasympathetic nervous system, and rest. When you take this moment of mindfulness, a solution may come on how to manage the task or problem you were worrying about a second before more efficiently or enjoyably. Maybe the solution is to ask for help or turn it over to someone else. If you are in the middle of doing something, stepping out of your current state for just five to ten minutes may feel like an inconvenience, but it can often give perspective and actually result in saving you time and energy in the end, not to mention restore your enteric nervous system back into balance.

Here are four steps I give when leading guided meditation for a group or individual. I use these same steps for myself when under stress. Whether you practice these steps in the middle of an activity or during downtime, they can help you take a step back from a stressful situation and reconnect inwardly with what you truly need in the moment, rather than reach for something sweet or another distraction.

1. Be fully present with what you are feeling right now, bringing focus to your senses and into the present (sight, sounds, feeling).
2. Watch your breath move at its own natural pace—in through the nose, filling the lungs, and releasing back out into the space in front of the face. Release any control over your breathing by allowing the feeling of surrender to what is happening in the present moment.
3. Every time you feel your to-do list, fears, worries, or any other anxiety-provoking thought coming in to pull your attention away from your breath, imagine holding that thought in your hands and placing it in a stream flowing in front of you. Release it into the water and watch it float downstream, getting farther away until you can no longer see it. Do this with every fear and worry that comes up, until you are free to relax into the movement of your breath, feeling the breath fully, moving in and out, in and out.
4. Check in with your heart and send yourself a lifeline. Acknowledge any feelings present, whether they are feelings of connection and gratitude, or feelings of loneliness, criticism, or fear. Just allow whatever comes to your awareness to be there, without judgment or pretense. As you send loving compassion to yourself for any perceived weaknesses or mistakes, find a quality or mantra to meditate on that brings you strength. One of my favorites during stressful and often frustrating moments with my daughter is: *I'm a good and loving mother.* If you're stressed at work, maybe yours is something more like: *I am capable and savvy at what I do,* or *I have loving support from those around me.*

MAKE YOUR OWN MANTRA

When I first started meditating, I found it to be relaxing in a way like other monotonous activities—cooking dinner, folding laundry, doing light hatha-style yoga, or going for a walk. It helped me get my mind off my troubles, but it also sometimes felt a bit like a chore that I had to get through. I found it helpful to use a mantra to clear my mind, especially in the first five to ten minutes of my meditation. Mantras and counting prayer beads are commonly used in the Sufi, Buddhist, and Hindu practices of meditation. By focusing on one word, sound, or phrase over and over, we train our mind to weed out our worries and fears and let go of the incessant monkey-chatter in our mind. Slowly, this peripheral noise quiets down and we can sit in a more centered, tuned-in frequency with our bodies. The trick is to continually come back to that word, that phrase, or our breath even as our mind tries to think about our to-do list, latest life drama, or other matter. I often choose a phrase based on how I am feeling in the moment and say it either in my head or softly out loud at a slow pace in line with my breath, on each exhale. If I am feeling tight and closed off, I'll choose a mantra like *openness*. If I'm feeling scared or unsafe, I'll tell myself, *You are safe from harm*, or *You are surrounded in safety and love*. By saying it on an exhale, I imagine that these phrases are settling into my being and becoming a part of me, replacing my fears and worries.

All day long we may try to appear happy to the world around us, while inside we may be feeling a mixture of fear, anger, desire, jealousy, confusion, shame, empathy, grief, or overwhelm as well. Those feelings are equally valid and part of our human experience just as much as contentment. It may seem cliché, but creating your own mantra to validate your inner world and then practicing mantra meditation during your day, even for just ten to twenty minutes, can help bring much-needed compassionate attention on the overall state of your body and nervous system, which often includes all these more challenging emotions. By releasing into whatever feelings are "up" for you in the moment and recognizing with deep acceptance the true state of your emotions, it is much easier to relax into the present moment, rather than continuing to put up resistance to any undesirable feelings.

To this day I continue to come back to my mantras and breathe, both during and outside of my meditation practice, whenever my mind starts to wander down a path that is causing me pain and anxiety. Sometimes it's not even until I find myself meditating on a mantra I've done in the past that I fully acknowledge the true state of my physical being. Just taking five to twenty minutes to step out of whatever I am thinking about and step back into my body by doing mindful yoga stretches or sitting in a mantra meditation can change my outlook like a refresh button, allowing me to start my day over coming from a more authentic perspective and understanding within.

When we get stuck in a strong emotional state, our feelings may become so intense we feel the need to "shut them off" to better cope with the situation. Yet by shutting off our emotions, we lose all the good ones too and disconnect from the part of us that makes life worth living. If we stay in this state of disconnect for too long, we may enter deeper and deeper into depression, losing touch with the things we love in life. Whenever I'm going through a big change in my life or other stressful event and feel the familiar overwhelming sense of fear in my chest, to avoid getting stuck long-term in a fearful rut, so to speak, I try every day to refocus my mind on my mantras and breathing naturally to bring me back into my body. Even for just twenty minutes or so, if that's all the time I have. I find this mantra practice to be helpful in developing a focused, yet relaxed, physical state both during and outside my meditation. With each exhale, I say the mantra in my head or out loud to refocus my mind and realign my heart into connection with my body's natural state. By first becoming present with the true state of my body and recognizing this to be my reality at that moment, it's not only easier and more enjoyable to meditate, it's also easier and more enjoyable to live life. The present state of our body and nervous system may be hard to look at, and may not be who we want to be—like a big ol' pot of stew with a little of everything all mixed together—but it's who we are in this moment, and it's beautiful, regardless of what leftover veggies may have been tossed in. This practice of connecting with our physical body is magical and creates more genuine interactions with the world around us, allowing us to fully appreciate and take in the experiences and people in our lives. Our authentic self includes all of our failure, loss, pain, and grief, and that's part of what makes us who we are.

When I was living in Oregon, I had the opportunity to study a prayer-based form of meditation in a community of Sufis practicing in Northern California. In this mystical branch of Islam, the focus is not on reading the Koran, but rather connecting with one's heart to bring about loving kindness toward oneself and others. As is the case with many mystical spiritual transitions, the core of the practice is self-transformation. The Sufis have a word they use to describe the inner constitution, or driving force, pushing us to go beyond our comfort zone and courageously pursue our highest aspirations—which requires us to transform who we think we are. They call this state *himma*.

In one word they marry all the "Stages of Change," defined in the field of behavioral psychology as the steps toward changing an old habit or ingraining a new behavior into one's life. These stages include the state of setting a goal, of having the will to take action, letting go of inhibiting mind-sets, and pushing through fears or setbacks that get in the way of achieving that goal. I don't know if we have such a powerful word in the English language to describe this intrinsically human state. The Buddhist terminology most similar to this would be *bodhicitta*, or the volition toward changing for good and helping others to the same end as one's own purpose on earth. The Sufis have a word for this inner driving force—at least according to some traditions—because they see *himma* as the essence of the human being, our inner, most true nature. To get in touch with one's *himma*, one must declutter the mind and open the heart. While learning this form of Sufi mantra meditation, I realized that for me to reach a state of such clear mind-set and confidence in pursuit of my goals, I needed to declutter my mind and develop more faith in my innate ability to love, first and foremost, myself.

Developing trust in my ability to care for myself and learning how to recognize the true state my body was in, without judgment, gave me permission to release many of the fears and worries that I'd been carrying around since childhood. I realized that when I was in a self-critical mode, my heart was closed off. I then perceived that lack of compassionate connection I was experiencing in myself, from my family and friends, and even from the world around me.

TUNING IN TO YOUR BODY

You can practice bringing this kind of mindful, loving attention toward your own body in any moment, while walking, sitting at your desk, or at home. Start by simply bringing your undivided attention to what your body is seeing, hearing, smelling, and feeling right in the moment. This effort could include the feeling of your feet on the ground as you go for a walk, the feeling of your breath as you sit quietly, or even a strong physical sensation in your body. The key is to keep your focus on just one sensory object for an extended period of time. If you are focusing on a feeling in your stomach and you notice you are thinking about something else, bring your attention back to your stomach and imagine your breath flowing and infusing that part of your body with oxygen. If you have some distracting thoughts, it is okay to notice them. Maybe they are important to acknowledge for a moment, but then come back to your meditation object. If you feel a strong emotion arise, don't push it away; it's okay to sit with it and let that feeling be your meditation object for a while, eventually bringing your mind back to your breath. Maybe you notice a pain in your upper shoulder while sitting. Rather than wincing and trying to ignore this pain, bring loving kindness to your shoulder, as if you were asking it, *What have you been carrying around all day, dear shoulder? I'm here to listen to you.* If you haven't already, eventually tune in to your gut and notice what's happening there. Continue to check in with different parts of your body, asking the same questions. See if you can listen to each specific part of your body and hear what it has to say.

This kind of mindfulness practice can drastically begin to affect how we view and treat our own body, impacting both our food choices and our awareness of activities we do all day long. A few years ago, after recently renewing my commitment to my daily meditation practice, I was strolling down my usual route toward a café in the South End of Boston. The front of each apartment was identically decorated with an ascending fairy tale–like staircase leading to a double-door entrance. Lush green garden landscaping separated each staircase, and every twenty yards or so, a grand stone fountain sat in the middle of the street, the top of each just barely reaching the bending branches of the looming trees lining the street. Whether planned or unintentional, these fountains created the perfect substitute speed bumps, forcing cars to maneuver around the large structures with agility and care. This design allowed the street to remain separate and quiet, compared to the busy traffic a few blocks away, and created a calm, peaceful environment, almost silent but for the birds chirping overhead and the echo of my steps.

Suddenly, I had the desire to start a walking meditation. Bringing my focus to my steps on the uneven stone sidewalk, I trekked down the cobblestone streets lined with brownish redbrick apartments. My thinking pattern up to this moment had been caught in its habitual momentum, and I wasn't paying much attention to most of the thoughts, feelings, and underlying beliefs streaming through my mind. Yet a change in awareness occurred as I started to bring my attention to my steps, one by one, as I walked down the street. I soon found my attention diverted from the constant back chatter in my head, and I began to feel more present in my body. Despite having walked down this street countless times before, it was as if I was seeing my surroundings for the first time. The colors became more vivid and seemed to pulse with life. My body breathed a sigh of relief, finally getting a break from the steady stream of worried thoughts flowing through my mind toward the vast and unknown outlets in the far reaches of my brain. After about fifteen minutes, I seemed to enter a more simple and carefree state of existence. Free of analysis, rational thinking, and pro versus con debates in my mind, I started to feel the stress of everyday life simply melting away. In this moment I realized that a second ago I hadn't even been conscious of this back chatter. Only in noticing its absence did I become fully aware of its almost constant presence.

Arriving at the café, I felt grateful that I was able to walk the eight blocks rather than taking the bus. As I stepped inside I was bombarded by tempting sweets. I tried to maintain my newfound centered mind-set, but started to feel distracted. Desperately I searched the shelves behind the counter for something to give me the energy I needed without sugar's highs and lows. However, the rows were only lined with buttery baked goods, chocolates, and savory pies. The drink menu was no better: coffee, coffee with milk, coffee with cream, and coffee with flavored sugar, syrup, and cream, or tea. Connecting with the mindfulness I had worked on achieving through my walking meditation, I picked out a lightly caffeinated green tea and a hearty vegetable soup before ducking out of the temptation zone.

It's truly amazing how life transforms when we make even the smallest choices from a more connected place. Next time you're walking to buy lunch or get a snack, try doing a walking mediation on the way there, even if just for a few minutes. Focus on the feeling of your steps as each foot hits the ground, the things you see in your surroundings, or the sounds you hear. Once you reach your destination, notice if it's easier to make a mindful decision on what to eat, and how you feel about what you chose.

CULTIVATING A MINDFUL EATING PRACTICE

Mindful eating develops the awareness of what you are about to put into your body, your one true home. Where did it come from? Why are you eating it? How do you feel about eating it? As you stay with your senses, you'll start to notice what the food actually tastes like and what the microbes in your body are telling you as soon as a bite hits your tongue. When you are fully present with your body and mind while eating, you become aware of your actual relationship with food, or even with that particular food. Then you can decide how to choose intentionally for your well-being.

Finding a cohesive balance in our gut requires a mindful practice of tuning in and noticing how our body and belly feel after eating a meal. Do you feel tired and groggy, or simply relaxed and satisfied? Do you feel pleasantly full, uncomfortably stuffed, or maybe bloated? Do you feel like your body is energized by the food you ate, or is your meal sitting like a rock in your stomach—not easily digestible by your body? Notice your mind too. Does it feel more awake and focused after the meal, or sleepy and scattered? Notice your behaviors after eating certain foods. Do you feel like pursuing a new project, or sitting around watching TV?

Starting to pay close attention to how your body responds to the food you are eating is a mindfulness practice in and of itself. This practice requires you to take space from your to-do list—allowing a moment to check in with yourself prior to, during, and after eating a meal—and take note of which foods you think may have caused any positive or negative aftereffects. When we begin to choose foods with intention—*I want to have more energy, feel satisfied, relaxed, and comfortable in my body, while maintaining a clear mind and feeling focused in my life*—our choices may change dramatically, even without designing a meal plan for the week or trying to force ourselves into a new health regimen. Allow yourself to savor and enjoy the process of choosing your foods, at least once a day to start. If there is one meal a day where you often eat alone, this time presents the perfect opportunity to bring in a mindful eating practice.

Another effective mindful eating practice is counting the number of times I chew each bite, making sure it's at least thirty times. Thoroughly chewing your food not only increases how satisfied you feel after you eat, but also helps you taste and appreciate all the subtle flavors and textures in the meal. Chewing longer also increases the digestive juices in your stomach so that your digestive tract is more ready to receive your food after you swallow and helps your body absorb more of the nutrients. Not to mention you're manually doing more of the digesting before the food enters your stomach, which will lead to fewer digestive problems such as feelings of gas and bloat. Even if you only count the number of times you chew each bite for five minutes, you will reap these benefits, so it's worth a try!

Practicing Mindful Eating

When you first start a mindful eating practice—even if you can only practice at one meal a week to start—it's best to either practice alone or with others who will respect your silence. You can also begin this practice while preparing your meal, rather than waiting until you are seated in front of your food. I've found that even having the intention to do this practice while eating helps me prepare my food with fresh, new intentions for my vitality and health. *Am I tired and in a rush, so my intention is just to eat as quickly as possible? Or am I relaxed and feeling creative, wanting to experiment with something new?*

As you prepare to eat in a private space, tune in to the sounds in your surroundings. Maybe it's just the silence of the room broken by the gentle clanking of your plate and silverware. Or, if you're outside with the sounds of nature, maybe you hear the trees whistling or a dog barking in the distance. Whatever your environment, take it in for a moment before picking up your fork and spoon. After about a minute, prepare for your first bite. Pause right before placing a bite of food into your mouth and notice how the smells of the food make you feel. Ask yourself how you anticipate feeling after this meal, and set your intention for how you want to feel: *I want to feel satisfied but not overly full, energized and relaxed.*

Once you start eating, really taste your food. If you find it difficult to eat slowly, count your chews, up to thirty or forty chews, before swallowing the first five bites. Eat one piece of food at a time and really savor it. Notice the sensory experience before taking the bite, taste it fully while chewing, and then experience the lingering flavors after swallowing. Like all things in life, taking a moment to be fully present with an experience, to savor and reflect, will bring meaning and insight to the situation.

ADDITIONAL MINDFULNESS RESOURCES

Smartphone Apps

- Mindfulness Coach (iOS)
- Calm (iOS and Android)
- 10 Percent Happier (iOS and Android)
- Buddhify (iOS)
- Headspace (iOS and Android)
- Insight Timer (iOS and Android)
- Mindi (iOS)
- The Smiling Mind (iOS and Android)
- The Mindfulness App (iOS and Android)
- Zen Timer

Websites

- UCLA Mindful Awareness Research Center, Free Guided Meditations: http://marc.ucla.edu
- Ronald Siegel, PsyD., Free Mindfulness Meditations: http://www.mindfulness-solution.com
- Palouse Mindfulness: http://palousemindfulness.com
- Dharma Seed: http://www.dharmaseed.org

Books

- *Mindfulness in Plain English* by Bhante Gunnaratana
- *Mindfulness, Bliss, and Beyond* by Ajahn Brahmavamso (this one is funny, too)
- *Work: How to Find Joy and Meaning in Each Hour of the Day* by Thich Nhat Hanh

TAKEAWAYS

- Cortisol is a hormone created by our adrenal glands to help us deal with stress. An increase in this stress hormone can cause salt and sugar cravings and affect digestion.
- In creating cortisol, our body uses up our stores of vitamins D, B5, B6, B12, and C, affecting our body's ability to fight off viruses and get good-quality sleep. High cortisol also weakens the adrenal glands and disrupts our ability to make other hormones, leading to hormonal imbalance (think serotonin, the mood hormone). This imbalance can increase our chances of developing depression and anxiety.
- Our mental state can often be the culprit triggering physical symptoms of stress. Meditation is a proven way to reduce stress by reprogramming our mind to relax and take a step back from our anxiety and overwhelm.
- Mindfulness is our heartfelt, nonjudgmental awareness of experiences in the present moment. It is a way to reconnect with our innermost feelings and develop an awareness of underlying fears and emotions that may be causing stress.
- Mindfulness-Based Stress Reduction (MBSR) is a proven therapy to reduce stress. In regularly practicing meditation and mindfulness skills, you can learn how to reconnect with yourself and be more mindful in every choice you make.
- Mindful eating is a practice that brings awareness to our relationship with food and our body and helps us eat in a way that practices self-care.

· *6* ·

What Are Sugary Foods, Exactly?

$\mathcal{N}$ow it's time to learn how to identify hidden sugars in your food so you know which foods are feeding the pathogenic flora in your gut. Once you stop feeding the pathogenic flora, it becomes easier to distinguish sugar cravings for what they are—a gut microbial imbalance that needs to be brought back in balance. A common misconception about limiting sugary foods is the myth that only added sugar needs to be removed or limited in the diet to detox the liver, reduce inflammation, restore the microbiome, and balance blood sugar, when in fact there are many other foods that contain sugars or refined carbohydrates and act similar to sugar thus having a detrimental effect on our microbial balance, such as bread, milk, fruit juice, and beer, wine, and other alcoholic drinks. Research suggests that drinking alcohol can increase gut permeability, ultimately creating an imbalance of gut bacteria—termed gut dysbiosis.[1, 2] If we are avoiding added sugars but drinking a glass of wine every night, this can affect our microbiome and liver to a comparable degree. For this reason refined carbs, juices, and alcoholic drinks need to be kept to a minimum or removed completely during your sugar detox if you want to restore balance to your gut and overall health.

Alcohol will be covered more in depth in chapter 8. For now, suffice it to say that even small amounts will hinder the desired, natural detox process and rebalancing of the microbial strains in your gut. After a month, if you feel ready you can start to add small amounts of alcohol very carefully, staying attuned to symptoms of disrupted flora and *Candida* growth. Although most forms of distilled alcohol, such as whiskey, bourbon, vodka, tequila, and gin, don't contain any sugar unless they are an ingredient in mixed drinks, they can further inhibit a sugar detox by disrupting your body's detox pathways and place an added burden on the liver.

IS THERE SUCH A THING
AS *HEALTHY* SUGAR HABITS?

Most nutritionists and doctors will tell you that it's fine to eat small amounts of sugar or other high-glycemic foods regularly. What they rarely say, however, is what constitutes a "safe" amount in today's world. In other words, how much is really too much? Research shows eating one hundred grams of sugar or refined carbs—roughly equivalent to twenty-four ounces of soda—inhibits the ability of white blood cells to engulf and destroy harmful microorganisms and particles that are foreign to the body, thereby considerably weakening the immune system.[3] By comparison, a slice of white bread contains roughly fifteen grams of refined carbohydrates, so a sandwich would contain roughly thirty grams. This impairment of immune function begins within thirty minutes after sugar is ingested and lasts for more than five hours afterward. Two hours after consuming 50–100 grams of a high-glycemic food—at the height of immune suppression—our white blood cell function is diminished by 50 percent! When white blood cells are impaired, the body's overall immune response is greatly depressed and greatly increases our chances of catching a cold or infection. On the flip side, consuming fibrous prebiotics has the opposite effect, enhancing our immune function.[4]

Judging from the research, we want to avoid refined carbohydrates as much as possible, and it's safe to say that consuming anywhere between fifty to one hundred grams of refined carbohydrates (bread, sugar, soda, juice, beer, or wine) in a single day is too much, and especially if you are trying to detox your body of sugar or want to avoid getting sick during flu season, or already feel a cold coming on! Over 50 grams of refined carbohydrates will most definitely suppress your immune system, further increasing your chances of becoming sick and hampering your body's ability to fight pathogenic bacteria.

SUGAR DETOX PHASE I: SUGAR

Your first step in restoring microbial balance is to identify how much sugar is in the most common foods in your diet, and then to consume no more than ten grams of refined sugars per day—not including whole fruits or whole-fat dairy products. Fruit juice and milk, however, do count toward your ten grams a day. Not only do these drinks contain fructose, lactose, and sucrose, but they are refined liquid carbohydrates that, similar to sugar, cause a spike in blood sugar and disrupt insulin levels. Whole milk is by far the best choice, if you are going to drink milk, yet all forms of cow's milk count toward your ten grams a day due to their high lactose content and its effect on insulin levels, which we'll get into later in chapter 8: "Sugar Incognito." If you're not sure how much sugar is in milk or juice, check the label—it is listed on every carton and bottle. Milk and fruit juice list their sugar content on the label, which is lumped into the "Total Sugars" row along with any added sugars. If you only see whole fruit listed on a nutrition label and no added sugars, you're in the clear. However, if 100 percent fruit juice is an ingredient in a healthy food, then count it toward your ten grams. If this sounds confusing, just remember that all products that count toward your ten grams will have a label on them, and whole fruits and vegetables don't count toward your ten grams. Just be sure you're reading the labels on everything you eat for the sugar content and you will be in the clear!

The only exception to this rule is unsweetened whole-fat dairy products like yogurt, kefir, and aged cheeses that list enzymes and probiotics on the ingredient label. These products do contain a small amount of natural sugars, but since they have enzymes, probiotics, and loads of healthy fats—as long as you don't have an allergy to dairy—they will support the rebalancing of your gut and blood sugar, not contribute to it. Butter is one dairy product you definitely don't have to worry about at all, as it doesn't contain any natural sugars. All forms of milk found in the grocery store will not help your gut flora and should be avoided. If you can find cultured or unpasteurized whole milk at a local farm, this would count as an exception along with yogurt and other whole-fat cultured milk products due to their high content of enzymes and probiotics.

As far as sweeteners go, I highly encourage you to include one teaspoon of molasses or raw honey (equivalent to about five grams of sugar) in your daily ten grams a day sugar detox phase to increase the alkalinity of the body and ward off illness. Monk fruit extract, stevia extract, organic coconut sugar, and lucuma fruit are additional all-natural sweeteners that I'd recommend using over cane sugar. These superfood sweeteners contain high concentrations of essential minerals, antioxidants, and other nutrients that make them alkaline and safe for our microflora, unlike most other sweeteners. Raw honey in particular is the only sweetener that actually serves as a health-promoting food for the beneficial flora in our gut. Blackstrap molasses contains high amounts of iron, calcium, magnesium, vitamin B6, and selenium, which help us manage stress, balance our hormones, and stabilize blood sugar levels. All these sweeteners are low-glycemic, safe for your gut flora, and delicious sugar substitutes.

Monk fruit and stevia extract contain no sugar at all, so you don't have to worry about them counting toward your ten grams.

Wondering what ten grams of sugar looks like? Ten grams of sugar is about equivalent to one-half cup of sweetened granola, one-quarter of a bar of dark chocolate, one measuring cup of skim milk, or two teaspoons of honey. Be aware of salad dressings, sauces, and marinades with hidden sugar content. Most commercial ketchup has up to six grams of high-fructose corn syrup per tablespoon, so make sure to choose the organic, sugar-free ketchup on the shelf. If you're a soda lover, watch out. An eight- to twelve-ounce can of soda can have up to forty to fifty grams of refined sugar!

If you don't have any sensitivities to dairy and want to keep dairy in your diet during this phase, organic, whole-fat dairy such as no-sugar-added whole-fat yogurt or aged cheeses are best. If you want to include milk, remember it counts toward your ten grams a day and whole-fat is best because the fat content helps us absorb the fat-soluble vitamins A and D found in milk—with the added benefit of helping to curb the lactose sugar spike. If the milk is from a local grass-fed dairy farm and uses low-heat pasteurization or no pasteurization, this is most ideal, as it will still contain natural enzymes including phosphatase, amylase, and lactase, which aid digestion and absorption of nutrients.

NEW NUTRITION LABEL
WITH "ADDED SUGAR" COLUMN

The Federal Drug Administration has issued a new nutrition label, and over the next few years, companies will be required to print nutrition labels with a new "Added Sugar" column located beneath the "Total Sugars" (see Figure 6.1). Typical added sugars include corn syrup, sucrose, concentrated fruit juice, fructose, brown sugar, cane sugar, conventional honey, and so forth. The total sugars column includes both added sugars, such as honey or cane sugar, and any natural sugars found in the food, such as lactose in milk or fructose in whole fruit juice or jam products. Pay attention to how many grams of natural sugar and added sugar there are per serving and how large or small the serving size. (See Table 6.1.) Once you identify the biggest sugar offenders in your own diet, look for new non-sugar or natural alternatives to swap in.

To find out exactly what types of sugars a product contains, make sure to read the list of ingredients under the "Nutrition Facts."

Nutrition Facts

8 servings per container
Serving size   2/3 cup (55g)

Amount per 2/3 cup

Calories   230

% DV*	
12%	**Total Fat** 8g
5%	Saturated Fat 1g
	Trans Fat 0g
0%	**Cholesterol** 0mg
7%	**Sodium** 160mg
12%	**Total Carbs** 37g
14%	Dietary Fiber 4g
	Sugars 1g
	Added Sugars 0g
	Protein 3g
10%	Vitamin D 2mcg
20%	Calcium 260mg
45%	Iron 8mg
5%	Potassium 235mg

* Footnote on Daily Values (DV) and calories reference to be inserted here.

Figure 6.1. New Nutrition Label with "Added Sugar" Column

Here's a list of products where added sugars are typically found:

- Condiments and sauces such as ketchup, barbecue and teriyaki sauce, plum sauce and other Asian sauces
- Low-fat or fat-free salad dressings and marinades
- Dips and spreads
- Side dishes from the supermarket deli (coleslaw, macaroni)
- Canned biscuits and pizza dough
- Yogurt
- Takeout, especially pizza and Chinese food

Added sugars in the freezer:

- Frozen entrées (low calorie or otherwise)
- Processed meats (sausage, hot dogs)
- Frozen veggies prepared with sauces
- Breakfast sandwiches
- Mini pizza, bagels, pizza rolls, pocket sandwiches
- Frozen bread and rolls
- Potpies

Added sugars in the pantry:

- Pasta sauce
- Instant or flavored oatmeal
- Granola, fruit and grain bars (whole grain varieties as well)
- Cereal bars
- Sweetened cornbread mix
- Whole grain cold cereals
- Bread, whole grain/white/pita
- Baked beans
- Trail mix
- Whole grain crackers
- English muffins, bagels
- Tortilla wraps

Table 6.1. Approximate Sugar Content of Common Foods

Food/Drink	Approximate Sugar (Grams)
Grape or Apple Juice (unsweetened), 1 cup	35 grams
Sweet and Sour Chicken (1 frozen entrée)	16 grams
Blueberry Muffin	15.5 grams
Granola, 1/2 cup	13 grams
Fast-Food Double Cheeseburger	9 grams
Spaghetti Sauce, 1/2 cup	7 grams
Snack Pack Pudding Cup	20 grams
Bottled Green Tea	30–50 grams
Bottled Iced Tea	45–60 grams
Sweetened Yogurt	2–30 grams
Frozen Breakfast Waffles	16 grams

OUT OF SIGHT, OUT OF MIND?

Maybe you're now wondering, *If sugar is so addictive and unhealthy, then why allow even ten grams a day*? Our primary goal during this detox phase is to create a sustainable alkaline state in your body that allows your microflora to recalibrate and your liver to detox from sugar's effects, without creating the "forbidden-fruit" syndrome. Many of us have tried those diets where we deprive ourselves of something we love for a certain amount of time, and then as soon as we reach the end, or perhaps even beforehand, we binge on the foods we long for—making us feel even worse about ourselves than when we started. If you've ever done a diet like this, you know that most of the time these diets result in gaining all the weight back, and then some! The key difference between a long-term plan for success and a short-term diet lies in the important marker that you don't feel completely deprived at any point during this phase. By allowing a small amount of sugar from the beginning, it will be easier to continue to keep sugar to a minimum, even after this first phase is over. A few people I've coached over the years have chosen to just cut out sugar altogether during this phase, rather than having the ten grams of sugar a day, even if this is slightly more difficult for them to do. But most folks I've worked with who are trying to break a long-term sugar habit find that cutting it out completely leaves them feeling denied of something they love, and are more likely to go back to their old sugar habits after the first detox is over.

When we feel completely deprived of anything, it can often backfire and create an increased desire. Our imagination can run wild over how delicious our favorite food would taste, *if only, if only*—thus making it inevitable we will cheat or revert back to old habits after the diet is over, or reach for an equally unhealthy alternative such as alcohol to curb sugar cravings. If you strive only for perfection, you are setting yourself up for failure. Whenever we try to be perfect, failure to do so can trigger self-shaming, which has been scientifically linked with depression and weight gain. Self-criticism is simply not allowed. If you must cheat, cheat! Then, congratulate yourself for making it as far as you did, even if it was only two or three days. After patting yourself on the back for a successful first attempt, just start the process over again—but whatever you do, don't let your self-talk revert to criticism. In both my personal experience and my practice coaching individuals over the years, this sort of mental spiral often leads to short-term and long-term bingeing, a perceived sense of failure, and a reversion back to old habits. A combination of the deprivation effect and self-criticism is why most typical dieters gain back more weight after finishing their diet, rendering the diet harmful rather than helpful. Indeed, some diets can actually be a cause for weight *gain* rather than weight loss in the end.

Research supports the approach of allowing a small amount of the favored food while tackling sugar habits. According to researchers in the Department of Psychology at Princeton University, when one group of rats that had been given a consistent intake of sugar water followed by two weeks of abstinence was compared to another group of rats that had been given thirty minutes daily access to sugar water, the rats that were forced to abstain completely experienced increased intake and a "deprivation effect," which has been scientifically linked to drug abuse in other rat studies.[5] Of course, we are not rats, but when we allow ourselves just a bite of something every once in a while, it helps to at least minimize, if not eliminate, the feeling of loss and avoid the deprivation effect and negative self-criticism spiral.

This approach also encourages discretion when "choosing your poisons," so to speak. Maybe you forgo the plate of cookies at work, knowing that you have some dark chocolate waiting for you at home later that night. Maybe your daily breakfast bar is healthy but happens to contain seven grams of sugar, which then becomes your one allowance during this phase. This way you can keep some of your favorite things without overdoing it. It also helps us to truly appreciate treats when we do have them, without getting caught up in worrying about them.

Avoiding pitfalls when you're trying to stick to ten grams of added sugar a day requires knowledge and reduced temptation. Knowing how much added sugar is in foods is vital if you want to reduce or eliminate refined sugar. (See Table 6.2.) Remove temptation by doing a full sweep of all sugar at home and work. Let no secret stashes remain! Empty out your desk drawer at work and give your sweets away to your coworkers. If you don't want to throw stuff away at home, give them to a neighbor. Whatever you do, don't rely completely on willpower during the course of your sugar detox. As I mentioned earlier, sugar is highly addictive and lights up the same areas of the brain as cocaine and tobacco. If you make it too easy to grab a sugary snack when a craving strikes, this easy availability may make it impossible to stick to the ten-gram daily limit.

Out in the world we're constantly bombarded with expectations to fit in, be productive, be social. However, home is the one environment we have control over. Home is our one place of refuge. This is your opportunity to transform your kitchen and home into a space that supports your health and well-being, rather than a temptation zone filled with guilt and regret. If your family objects to these changes, then you can invite them to keep their sweets somewhere else rather than in the kitchen or common areas, where they are not available to you. Clearing your house of sugar transforms your home into a safe space rather than a place of distraction and temptation.

Table 6.2.   List of Added Sugars to Keep Under Ten Grams a Day

• brown sugar	• brown rice syrup
• powdered sugar	• cane crystals
• corn syrup	• cane juice
• corn syrup solids	• caramel
• dextrose	• date sugar
• fructose	• evaporated cane juice
• high-fructose corn syrup (HFCS)	• fruit juice concentrates
• conventional honey	• glucose
• lactose	• invert sugar
• malt syrup	• maltose
• maltose	• malt syrup
• pancake syrup	• muscovado sugar
• raw sugar	• natural sugar
• sucrose	• rice bran syrup
• sugar	• rice syrup
• white granulated sugar	• sorghum syrup
• barley malt	• sucrose
• agave nectar	• syrup
• coconut syrup	• turbinado sugar
• beet sugar	• molasses

It's up to you to choose how long you think you need to cut out sugar to reset your system and break your sugar habits. I recommend one month to start. Research suggests it can take anywhere from twenty-one to sixty-six days to form new habits.[6] If a month sounds too daunting and you can't seem to stay away from sugar for even a day, then just start with a goal of two weeks. Once you reach that goal, you may feel ready to go for another two weeks. Remember, this is not a diet as much as it is a new way of eating—a way to reset your taste buds so they grow accustomed to the natural sweetness of fruits, vegetables, and whole grains and are satisfied with little to no refined sugars.

Our taste buds acclimate very quickly to the foods we are eating. Ten grams a day will reduce your sugar consumption enough to allow your liver to heal and reset your taste buds so that by the end of the reset period, foods that are naturally sweet, like yams sprinkled with a little butter and honey, apples, and other fruits, will satisfy your sweet tooth. If you're consistently eating refined sugars and then bite into an apple, it may register as sour rather than sweet because your sweet taste buds have acclimated to the intense sweetness of sugary foods that are not found in nature. Once we allow our body to detox and have new go-to sweets for when a cravings hits, it becomes easier and easier to avoid sugar. In fact, sugar starts to taste so intensely sweet that when the detox is over and you do eat a dessert on a special occasion, such as a wedding or birthday dinner, it may actually taste so unbearably sweet you won't want to eat it or may only want a couple of bites!

Reintroducing a small amount of sugar into your diet after this detox phase won't turn into a habit again as long as these foods remain out of your home, professional space, or other places you frequent on a daily basis. When they are readily and easily available, we are much more likely to fall back into our old patterns, compared to when they are relegated only to social get-togethers like dinner with friends or family gatherings. At that point, you will also have safe snack replacements handy in your work and home environments and go-to mindful eating exercises that you can turn to when the occasional craving hits.

After just one month, you will start to see and feel the physical benefits of increased energy, clearer skin, and weight loss and may want to continue another month. Most people I've introduced to this plan have found it easy to continue for two or three months. They no longer reach for sugar in their downtime. When they are looking for extra energy, they actually start to crave more fruits and vegetables. Once you've detoxed your body of sugar, rebooted your microbiome, and formed new habits around healthy sweets, you will find it much easier to tune in to your body's true signals and cravings, guiding you toward foods that promote self-care, rather than self-sabotage. You will feel more confident than ever before about your food choices. This newfound confidence will carry through to other decisions regarding where you prioritize your time, your attention, and your relationships. Trust me, the confidence high that comes as a result of reducing sugar during this phase is way better than any sugar high that sweets can offer you.

If you go a few grams over the allotted ten, or you're not exactly sure how many grams of sugar were in that small cookie or Chinese food you had at a party or restaurant, don't stress! Another goal of allowing ten grams a day during this phase is to make avoiding sugar as simple as possible so you don't need to overthink when making food choices. Let your tongue be your guide. If you taste an overly sweet sauce at a restaurant, just ballpark how much sugar you think might be in it. Most sweet or creamy sauces contain around five grams per half-cup serving of food.

If at any point you feel that sticking to ten grams of sugar in your diet is too hard to manage, I encourage you to allow more natural sweeteners into your diet, such as whole fruits, sweet root vegetables like yams and potatoes, stevia, monk fruit extract, and even a little extra molasses and raw honey. Try making whole fruit smoothies instead of drinking straight juice, or flavor your seltzer water with a splash of fruit juice rather than drinking soda.

But remember, if you start to increase your sugar consumption to twenty grams or more a day, your liver will become overburdened, which halts the sugar detox process, and you'll need to start over from scratch. So choose your foods carefully. If you start eating sugar regularly again, just press the reset button and start over until you've successfully reduced your sugar intake to approximately ten grams a day for one month. Whatever you do, don't give up! Keep trying until you've successfully cut it out for at least one month straight with no major cheats. This period is a time to not only reset your body, but also reset your life and what you used to think you were capable of.

SUGAR REPLACEMENTS

Once you're ready to replace the sugar in your diet with other foods that satisfy your sweet tooth, think creamy and fruity. Healthy full-fat or fiber-ful foods satisfy cravings without causing a blood sugar pendulum ride. Foods that have a natural sweetness to them such as sweet potatoes, dates, bananas, coconut milk, coconut cream, and nut butters like peanut butter, almond butter, cashew butter, and sunflower butter mixed with a little raw honey on an apple or whole grain toast are great on-the-go snacks to have handy. If you like to bake, try switching out your regular baking ingredients for muffins or cookies made with sweet overripe bananas, whole oatmeal, coconut cream, blended dates, nut butters, and almond flour. I've included a recipe for pumpkin muffins at the end of this chapter.

A creamy herbal tea with almond or coconut milk, sweetened with a pinch of monk fruit extract or raw honey, is a personal comfort food of mine—perfect in the evening when it's time to wind down and relax. In the morning or afternoon, green tea is the healthiest caffeinated stimulant to choose because of its epigallocatechin gallate (EGCG), which helps slow the breakdown of starches and sugars in the digestive tract, improving glucose tolerance and insulin sensitivity—effectively warding off mid-morning or mid-afternoon hunger pangs. Regular consumption of green tea has even been found to lower the risk of developing type 2 diabetes.[7, 8]

Sugar is not your enemy! Having a cookie, dark chocolate, or a bite of cake at a party is allowed, as long as you can limit it to your ten grams. There are also a number of sugars that contain nutrients and even prebiotics that are beneficial for your gut in small amounts. It is always better to include natural sugars from organic raw honey, maple syrup, coconut sugar or syrup, or molasses in place of refined table sugar as part of your ten grams a day. The difference between natural sweeteners like raw honey and molasses and refined cane sugar is that the chemical structure of refined cane sugar has been significantly changed, making it dangerous for our blood sugar as well as devoid of any real nutrition. Natural sugars have nutrients and are much less processed and refined so our body can digest them more slowly, allowing time to absorb all the vitamins and minerals they contain. Natural sugars are a better source of energy and less likely to be stored as fat. For example, coconut palm sugar also contains fiber, in this case inulin, a starchy prebiotic fiber that has a slightly lower insulin response than sucrose, or cane sugar, and is therefore lower on the glycemic index. Natural sugars are also safer for the microbiome because they often contain fat, fiber, and other vitamins and minerals along with sugars, making them nutritious and lower on the glycemic scale. Whole fruit is full of fiber, vitamins, and minerals, making it an ideal sugar to feed the beneficial flora in your microbiome. Just be wary of fruit juice, which may contain added table sugar, little to no fiber, and high amounts of fructose.

A personal favorite of mine is raw honey. Raw honey contains sugars in the form of dextrin, a starchy fiber that your gut flora love. Even though raw honey tastes extremely sweet, and can often be sweeter than table sugar, it has less than half the glycemic score of white sugar or processed honey, with lots of added health benefits. It's amazing how the manufacturing process of refined honey alone raises the glycemic score twice as high! Raw honey has a moderate score on the glycemic index, whereas most commercial honeys score in the high to dangerously high zone. Some research even shows that raw honey may help control blood sugar because it contains special sugars that actually promote healthy gut flora[9] rather than unhealthy microorganisms like *Candida*. Raw honey has even been found to contain six species of *lactobacilli* and four species of *bifidobacteria*, making it both a prebiotic and probiotic food. It also contains a small amount of a broad spectrum of vitamins and minerals including B6, thiamin, niacin, riboflavin, pantothenic acid and certain amino acids, calcium, copper, iron, magnesium, manganese, phosphorus, potassium, sodium, and zinc. Manganese is the most abundant mineral found in raw honey and coincidently plays a very helpful role in everyday blood sugar control. Manganese is needed to help enzymes with the metabolism of carbo-hydrates, amino acids, and cholesterol.[10]

Raw honey is also highly antimicrobial, which helps boost your immune system during the winter when you feel a cold coming on. I often recommend mixing raw honey with a little lemon and raw apple cider vinegar or herbal tea as an elixir to fight a cold or virus. There are a number of claims that consuming locally sourced raw honey, containing pollen from the same plants one is allergic to, can be useful for those suffering from seasonal allergies. In a 2011 randomized controlled pilot study of forty-four patients with a diagnosed birch pollen allergy, researchers in Finland found that patients who consumed birch pollen honey prior to pollen season had significantly better control of their symptoms compared to those on conventional allergy medication, and they had marginally better control of their symptoms compared to those using non-local honey.[11] Of course it can be tricky to find locally sourced raw honey, but if you suffer in the outdoors any time of year it may be worth checking with local farms in your area to see if they farm bees.

There are plenty of artificial sugar "substitutes" out there, but most of them are created in a laboratory where their chemical structures are completely changed from the original plant components. Because of this chemical reengi-neering, artificial sweeteners are completely foreign to your digestive tract and often just get processed through your liver as an unrecognizable, nonnutritious substance. Since we are trying to give our liver a break and support the health of our microbiome during this phase, we don't want to consume anything that will bog down our liver or reverse the sugar detox process. The list of side effects associated with some of the most common artificial sweeteners is long enough to scare most people away, if they have done their research. For ex-ample, erythritol, a common sweetener found in "sugar-free" foods, can cause side effects such as diarrhea, headache, and stomachache. These sorts of artificial sweeteners, often touting the fact they are calorie-free and help with blood sugar, are now suspected of actually leading to weight gain. There is increas-ingly convincing evidence that many of these sugar substitutes are likely to be stored as fat and are a potential cause of metabolic syndrome and obesity—even more so than sugar.[12] One study tested rats after they were fed artificially sweet-ened food. The study found that not only did the rats' metabolism slow down, but their appetite increased, causing them to consume more calories and gain more weight than rats fed sugar-sweetened food![13]

Stevia is a naturally sweet medicinal herb from the plant species *Stevia rebaudiana* naturally grown in Brazil and Paraguay, where it has been used for hundreds of years as both a sweetener and herbal remedy for stomach discom-fort. The plant gets its sweet taste from naturally occurring glycosides. In the process of making an all-natural stevia extract, these glycosides, along with other plant properties, are extracted from the stevia leaves by placing the plant in hot water. Stevia is a wonderful sugar replacement for your tea or coffee, but be careful because it can be up to 200 times sweeter than sugar. You only need a few drops in your tea or coffee to equal two teaspoons of sugar. I like the SweetLeaf brand because I know there are no additives and it is a natural extract of the plant. Similar to Stevia, monk fruit is also a natural plant extract with no effect on blood sugar. This sweetener has been used medicinally for centuries as an expectorant, cough remedy, and for help with respiratory ailments. It's also extremely high in powerful antioxidants called mogrosides and vitamin C. Studies have shown mogrosides inhibit reactive oxygen species and DNA oxidative damage, which helps fight free radicals and the development or progression of cancer.[14, 15, 16] Some sweeteners pretending to be all-natural stevia or monk fruit actually contain additional sugar-substitute ingredients like erythritol. Be wary of those. They must be avoided altogether if you are trying to detox your system and restore balance to your gut flora.

BIOME-FRIENDLY SNACKS

Now you'll need to find substitutes for your go-to sweet snacks that you just threw away. These will be the snacks and foods that you have nearby—handy in your desk drawer, handbag, backpack, or fridge. Before cutting out refined sugar, I used to grab a cookie, graham cracker, or sweetened popcorn when my afternoon or after-dinner slump hit. Because these snacks were organic or local brands, I felt like I was supporting the local economy and being healthy. By grabbing a high-glycemic food every time I had low blood sugar in between meals, not only was I training my body to crave this snack as a "pick-me-up," but I was also further destabilizing my blood sugar levels by consuming refined wheat sugar on an empty stomach. This set my blood sugar on an uphill climb, followed by the cliff drop to starvation and more sugar cravings, and further increased my habitual cravings for packaged baked goods to boot.

As I mentioned, at a previous job years back, I developed a habit of mindlessly eating sweetened popcorn, crackers, and other sweet snacks at my desk while working. I told myself I could stop at any time, but eventually realized I felt completely powerless to quit this habit. I had no idea why I was endlessly eating packaged snacks. I only craved them at work and often during the second part of the workday when the pressure to finish my projects would start to rise. It seemed I just needed a little extra "energy" to get me through the most stressful part of the day, and I felt the snacks provided that. However, when I put myself to the test and tried to cut them out of my day, I couldn't.

Once I realized I was engaging in an addictive-like behavior, I took a closer look. Reflecting and journaling on my compulsion to eat sugar at that time of day, I saw that it was a direct result of my rising stress levels. Looking even more deeply, I saw that the main cause of my stress was my own internal thought process. In my mind, I was my own worst critic. If I didn't finish my projects by the end of the day, I felt like a worthless and incapable worker. In reality, my boss was happy with my productivity, and I had plenty of time to finish the projects. Why was I pushing myself to finish them by the end of the day? Turns out, I was the one spinning the hamster wheel at hyper-speed, not my boss or anyone else.

Once you start grabbing new sugar-safe foods when your afternoon slump hits, your taste buds will begin to change, and you will actually start to crave these foods instead of your double mint-chocolate latte. To avoid sugar dips that trigger sugar cravings later in the day or evening, the key is to start your day with a high-fat, high-protein food and then respond to a sugar craving with a food high in fiber, fat, or protein, such as an apple with sugar-free almond or peanut butter, rather than processed, refined grains and sugar. Feel free to mix a little raw honey into the nut butter yourself! This snack is not only much more satisfying, but it soothes both your sweet tooth and low blood sugar in one hit. It's also packed full of vitamins and minerals and contains healthy fats that slow the sugar breakdown. This type of snack should hold you over another few hours or until the next full meal. Find some recipes and prepare your snacks ahead of time, such as in the beginning of the week, so you have them ready to go should a craving hit. A little planning will allow you to balance your sugar levels, boost your mood, and prevent you from overeating at your next meal, without any extra thought or effort.

Whole fruit like red grapes, melons, bananas, and pears will quench your sweet tooth and contain a lot less fructose than fruit juice or processed sugar, plus have the added prebiotic benefits of plant fiber. These are all great snacks to grab when you get a craving for candy, juice, or soda. Their fiber content and vitamin C will strengthen your immune system, and their natural sugar will satisfy your sweet tooth. For the purposes of the ten grams a day phase, you don't need to count whole fruit sugar. Just be sure to eat fruit as a complement to other protein- or fat-rich snacks to avoid a blood sugar spike, and in moderation if you suspect an overgrowth of pathogenic flora like *Candida*.

Examples of other good snack substitutes are:

- Lightly sweetened brown rice cakes lathered with my Miso-Nut Butter (see recipe).
- Trail mix with salty roasted cashews or other fatty nuts.

- Add a teaspoon of raw honey to sliced strawberries in the morning and by afternoon they will be a tasty, super-sweet topping to your favorite whole-fat, sugar-free yogurt.
- No fruit on hand? Have a small serving of whole-fat, probiotic-rich dairy, coconut, or almond-based yogurt with warmed raw honey and smashed pecans drizzled on top.
- Enjoy preparing my Go-Go Raw Chocolate Brownies (see recipe) for a healthy dose of sugar-free dark chocolate sweetened naturally by dates and nuts.

Miso-Nut Butter

This is a tasty, salty-sweet spread for whole grain rice crackers, apples, and other fruit or sprouted whole grain bread. Plus it contains live, active cultures and is loaded with vitamins and minerals.

Ingredients:

> 10 tablespoons salted, unsweetened roasted peanut or almond butter
> 6 tablespoons unpasteurized white or yellow miso
> 3 tablespoons raw honey

Directions:
Combine the peanut or almond butter, miso, and honey in a bowl and stir until smooth. Refrigerate until ready to use.

Go-Go Raw Chocolate Brownies

These are great to have on hand in the late afternoon when you need a burst of sweetness and energy with a healthy dose of fat, fiber, and carbohydrates. You can use any nut or seed combination you like in this snack, but I chose almonds mixed with walnuts because of almonds' crunchy texture and walnuts' high omega-3 fatty acid content and antioxidants.

Ingredients:

> 2 cups mix of roasted, salted almonds and walnuts, or other nut/seed mix of choice
> 2 cups soft Medjool dates, pitted
> 2 tablespoons coconut oil
> 3 tablespoons unsweetened raw cocoa powder and 2–3 tablespoons water

1 teaspoon sea salt
1 teaspoon vanilla extract
Optional: ⅓ cup sunflower butter or coconut butter
1 cup shredded unsweetened coconut

Directions:

1. In a large food processor fitted with an "S" blade, process the nut mixture until crumbly. Add dates, coconut oil, cocoa powder and water, sea salt, and vanilla (and sunflower butter or coconut butter, if using) and process again until a sticky, uniform batter is formed.
2. Scoop the dough into an 8-by-8 inch or similar size cake pan. Press batter into the bottom of the pan with a spatula to create an even layer. Sprinkle shredded unsweetened coconut on top. Place in the freezer or refrigerator to set for at least an hour before serving. Store in a sealed container in the fridge for up to a week, or in the freezer for an even longer shelf life.

Kale Chips with Nutritional Yeast

Ingredients:

Large bunch of kale
1 tablespoon olive oil
¼ teaspoon salt
Black pepper and nutritional yeast to taste

Directions:
Preheat oven to 350°F. Spray two baking trays with cooking spray. Wash kale, then remove center stem from each kale leaf and cut leaves into 2- to 3-inch-long pieces. Place kale in a large bowl, drizzle with olive oil, and sprinkle with salt, pepper, and nutritional yeast. Use your hands to massage the oil into the kale leaves. Evenly distribute kale onto baking sheets and bake until crispy, approximately 12 to 15 minutes.

Baked Yams with Cinnamon and Honey

Ingredients:

4 tablespoons butter
2 teaspoons lemon juice

1 tablespoon raw honey
1 teaspoon cinnamon
4 large yams or 3 pounds sweet potatoes, cut into roughly 2-inch pieces
Salt to taste

Directions:
Preheat oven to 350°F. In a small saucepan, heat butter and lemon juice just until butter melts, then stir in the raw honey and cinnamon and remove from heat (to preserve the enzymes in the honey). Place the cubed yams or sweet potatoes in a large bowl and drizzle the butter and honey mixture over top. Toss well to coat. Sprinkle with salt. Bake uncovered for about 30 to 35 minutes, stirring and turning with a spatula or wooden spoon every 10 minutes, until just fork-tender.

Sweet Coconut-Cream-Covered Fruit

Ingredients:
1 can cream of coconut or ½ cup coconut creamer
1 teaspoon raw honey
Dash of salt
Choice of berries or fruit such as strawberries, blueberries, and kiwi
Fresh mint leaves

Directions:
Scoop solidified coconut cream out of the can, leaving the coconut juice at the bottom. Place cream into a small individual-serving blender, small food processor, or a bowl and whisk or blend in the raw honey and salt, making sure not to over-blend or mixture will start to curdle. Chop up fruits and place into individual serving bowls. Drizzle coconut-honey mixture over top and place a mint leaf on top for garnish. Enjoy!

Pumpkin Paleo Muffins

Ingredients:

1 cup almond flour
½ cup coconut flour
1 teaspoon baking soda
¼ teaspoon salt
1 teaspoon pumpkin pie spice (nutmeg, cinnamon, cloves)
½ cup chopped pecans and/or walnuts, divided

2 eggs, lightly beaten
1 cup canned or fresh pumpkin puree
2 tablespoons butter, softened
1 teaspoon vanilla extract
¼ cup raw honey
Optional: ½ cup low-sugar carob or dark chocolate chips

Directions:
Preheat oven to 350°F and grease ten muffin cups. In a mixing bowl, whisk together almond flour, coconut flour, baking soda, salt, pumpkin pie spice, and ¼ cup nuts. Add eggs, pumpkin, softened butter, vanilla, and honey. Mix until smooth. Spoon into muffin cups and sprinkle remaining ¼ chopped pecans and/or walnuts on top. Bake for 20 to 25 minutes, until a toothpick comes out clean. Let cool, then enjoy!

WHAT ARE YOU *REALLY* CRAVING?

We all have our weak moments. These often strike at the end of a long workday, or after an argument with a friend or other stressful event. In these moments it's important to stay away from sugar and turn inward rather than reaching for a quick fix that will only serve to distract us temporarily. Free-style journaling and meditating in a quiet place are two of my favorite ways to process thoughts and feelings, and allow me to tap into what my inner cravings are really calling out for. Next time a craving for sugar strikes, instead of reaching for a sweet, grab a piece of paper and start writing—just to see what comes out. You'll be surprised by what you learn about yourself in the process of doing this exercise. Meditation gives us permission to sit with challenging feelings and create a safe space to observe those feelings without indulging them, or trying to stuff them away and forget about them. Sugar cravings present a perfect opportunity to sit and observe what feelings are up for you at the moment, allowing yourself to take a break and rest.

Maybe you realize that underneath your cravings for sugar, what you are really craving is love or appreciation for a job well-done. Maybe what you're really craving is simply to rest and find some quiet time to yourself. Once you get at the core of what your soul is craving, make a promise to yourself in that moment that you will honor that need without turning to sugar and ignoring this voice of truth. If you can't honor your inner calling at that moment, make a date in your calendar to take care of that need. Honoring that inner need may mean scheduling a twenty-minute nap later that day, a coffee date with a friend, or a soak in a relaxing evening bath when you get home from work. Even if you have to wait until after you put the kids to bed, find the time to honor the need your body and soul are really asking for.

TAKEAWAYS

- Deprivation diets don't work and often lead to a pendulum swing on the scale. In this phase, allow yourself a very small amount of sweets without going over ten grams a day.
- Replace sweeteners in your diet with foods and sweeteners that are naturally sweet, like whole fruits, raw honey, molasses, sweet potatoes, and so on.
- Raw honey tastes very sweet but does not spike the blood sugar to the same degree as white sugar—plus it contains vitamins, minerals, and healthy bacteria to populate our gut flora, and supports our immune system due to its microbial benefits.
- Stevia and monk fruit are both wonderful replacements for sugar since they have no effect on blood sugar and are natural plants, not a man-made sugar like other sugar alternatives.
- Remove all temptation at home and at work by doing a full sweep of your fridge, cabinets, and desk.
- Have healthy snacks on hand so you can grab those instead of a snack high in refined flour or sugar when a sweet cravings hits.
- Tune in to what your inner voice is trying to tell you through your sugar craving by journaling, meditation, yoga, or another relaxing activity alone.

· 7 ·

Wheat Gut

*W*hite refined flour is a simple carbohydrate easily converted to blood glucose. The classic example, Wonder Bread, has a GI of 73, located right above refined sugar, which holds a lower score of 65 on the glycemic scale. Pure glucose (GI of 100) is the highest point on the glycemic index and is used as a reference to all other foods. Waffles score 76, U.S. baguettes 95, whole wheat bread 69, pita bread 68, and rice cakes 82. All score higher than Coca-Cola at 63.[1] The more processed and refined the carbohydrate, the faster it breaks down in the body and the bigger the sugar rush. For this reason refined and processed grains such as bread and other baked goods can have a dangerous metabolic effect on blood sugar when consumed in high amounts or without sufficient fat, protein, and fiber. Pathogenic flora like *Candida* love to eat the abundance of glucose floating around as a result of eating nutrient-deficient carbohydrates that provide us with more glucose than our bodies actually need.

What about whole wheat or organic wheat? While it's true that whole wheat is less processed than regular wheat flours, in this age of genetically engineered hybrid wheat seeds, most wheat is a product of science regardless of whether it is whole wheat, organic, or not. Even the current USDA National Organic program permits cisgenic cell fusion hybrid seeds, which classifies them as genetically modified organisms (GMOs), in *organic* food production!

Processed, refined, and packaged foods were nonexistent in the human diet until very recently in our human trajectory. Only since the Industrial Revolution—the past 200 years of mankind's 6-million-year existence—have we had the technology to superheat milk and alcohol enough to kill most of the bacteria and all of the enzymes, and hyper-process grains, sugarcane, and corn until they are completely chemically separated from the original plant, creating an entirely new chemical structure. These isolated ingredients—wheat flour, sugar, corn syrup—then began to be used in thousands of common food products. Prior to the Industrial Revolution, all grains were ground with the use of stone milling tools, and they preserved the entire contents of the cereal grain, including the germ, bran, and endosperm—all the fibers our microflora benefit from. Seventy-two percent of our modern-day diet is composed of refined, processed foods (milk, cereals, refined sugars) that would not have been found less than a hundred years ago.[2] Evidence shows these foods lead to inflammation throughout the body and are a huge contributing factor in the spike of inflammatory-based health conditions in the United States such as food allergies, food sensitivities, childhood and adult-onset type 2 diabetes, obesity, and others we've seen on the rise in recent years.

Evolutionarily speaking, we would never have encountered such a high dose of refined carbohydrates in our ancient diet, and our bodies have not developed the ability to utilize this overflow of glucose in an efficient way. Instead, once these isolated sugars flood our bloodstream with more glucose than we need, our bodies shovel the excess sugar into fat cells, while bacteria and yeasts that feed on sugar flourish in our gut—not to mention the damage being done to our gut lining and bacteria composition. Together, the three masked musketeers—sugar, flour, and, as we'll see in the next chapter, many dairy products as well, work as a united front to wreak havoc in our digestive tract and destabilize our blood sugar.

Our microflora have not fared well throughout all the changes to the wheat crop over the last one hundred years. Researchers have discovered that the consumption of processed GMO wheat contributes to chronic inflammation and autoimmune diseases by increasing the permeability of the gut and initiating a pro-inflammatory immune response.[3] How has wheat become so toxic? To begin with, wheat is one of the most heavily subsidized crops in the United States, which means farmers get paid by the bushel rather than by consumer demand. The only way for farmers to make money with this arrangement is to produce, produce, produce—no matter the chemicals or techniques necessary. The result is the bug-resistant, hyper-growth-speed, hybridized, Monsanto GMO wheat of our modern day. The deamidation process of wheat, for example, edits the protein-coding sequence in plant mitochondria, making the wheat we buy today a water soluble product that can be mixed with any packaged food. Because of all these changes to the wheat crop, the wheat flour we consume is nowhere near the same as the wheat our ancestors ate, and has actually become foreign to our body and toxic to our microflora in many ways.

Rates of gluten intolerance, wheat sensitivities, and celiac disease in the United States are soaring. Modern-day gluten causes gut cells to release zonulin, a protein that can break apart the tight junctions holding your intestinal cell wall together.[4] When these cell walls lining your gut get broken apart by the proteins found in wheat, your gut can become "leaky," thus the popular terminology used among holistic health care providers, "leaky gut syndrome." When the cell wall is compromised, it allows everything from toxins, microbes, undigested food particles, and antibodies to escape from your intestines and travel through your bloodstream, accessing every other part of your body. This condition puts a huge strain on your kidneys and liver, backing up the detoxification process, as they are given the responsibility to clean all these unwanted particles out of your blood in addition to their usual job.

This increased permeability in the gut can further harm the body's absorption of key vitamins and nutrients and initiate an inflammatory immune response to clear out any food particles that may have breached the intestinal barrier. If you have a sensitivity to wheat, this could mean that some of the particles that escape through the lining in your gut could be the antibodies your body produced to attack the gluten in the first place. Now these antibodies are everywhere in your system and may end up attacking other organs and systems, including your skin, thyroid, or even brain, producing an inflammatory response in other parts of your body. This is likely one of the reasons gluten intolerance is so often found in people with inflammatory autoimmune conditions such as rheumatoid arthritis, type 1 diabetes, pernicious anemia, Grave's disease, Hashimoto's disease, Addison's disease, chronic active hepatitis, myasthenia gravis, lupus, Sjogren's syndrome, and scleroderma, to name a few.[5] These disorders share common genetic and immunological linkages with celiac disease.

As early as 1994, Harvard School of Public Health nutrition researchers found proof of the connection between high-glycemic foods and inflammation in their famous Nurses' Health Study. Beginning in 1984 researchers began to track the diet and health history of more than 75,000 women. At the start of the study, all nurses were given a clean bill of health. Ten years later, 761 had either been diagnosed or died from heart disease. When the Harvard researchers looked at the data, they found a strong connection between women eating a high-glycemic diet of refined carbohydrates such as wheat and those with inflammation and heart disease. Those who ate more of these types of foods doubled their risk for heart disease compared to those with diets only moderately high in carbs.

Another reason why wheat intolerance is on the rise is the effect that glyphosate, the primary chemical ingredient in Monsanto's weed-killer herbicide Roundup™, has on our delicate microbial ecosystem. Glyphosate use has risen exponentially since the introduction of Roundup Ready genetically engineered wheat and soy were introduced in 1996. Two-thirds of the total volume of glyphosate applied in the United States since 1974 has been sprayed just in the last ten years. Glyphosate is used on wheat crops to a much greater degree than other crops not only due to the sensitive nature of the plant and its high vulnerability to pests, but because Monsanto's seeds have been engineered to require Roundup™ to grow. A whopping 72 percent of the total glyphosate used on farms around the entire world is sprayed on U.S. crops.[6] We are one of the only countries in the Western Hemisphere to allow this pesticide to be sprayed without strict limitations on concentration or volume, and no other pesticide has come remotely close to such intensive widespread use.

Glyphosate was deemed safe for human consumption by the EPA as a result of a safety review performed by Monsanto over fifteen years ago.[7] The EPA is required to run a "registration review" of any given pesticide every fifteen years—which leaves a huge gap between scientific discoveries and understandings of how these chemical concentrations are affecting us today. Quite a lot has changed in the scientific understanding of pesticides and their effect on gut bacteria just in the last ten years, and we now know that glyphosate poses a huge potential threat to the health of our gut and detox pathways. There is mounting research on this chemical's harmful effects on gut bacteria, enzyme impairment, sulfate depletion, vitamin B12 and nutritional deficiencies, and kidney and thyroid disorders.[8, 9] Researchers at the Massachusetts Institute of Technology (MIT) published a paper in *Interdisciplinary Toxicology* explaining why the prevalence of gluten intolerance and celiac disease has increased dramatically over the last fifty years, right in line with the increased usage of glyphosate.[10, 11] We know celiac disease is associated with imbalances in gut bacteria, specifically a reduction in *lactobacilli* and *bifidobacteria*, which are known to be killed by glyphosate, while promoting an overgrowth of the pathogenic flora *C. difficile*. For thousands of years we have consumed a variety of traditional organic native wheat crops. It shouldn't come as a surprise that our sensitive gut microbes cannot survive once they come into contact with food treated with herbicides designed to kill superbugs. When examined in this light, it seems only natural that our bodies would react to this herbicide as a toxic foreign invader by amping up the immune system to get rid of it, thus triggering an inflammatory response in our bodies.

Fish exposed to glyphosate develop digestive problems that mirror the symptoms of celiac disease.[12] In both celiac disease and glyphosate exposure, we also see an impairment of cytochrome P450 enzymes, which play an important role in detoxifying environmental toxins, activating vitamin D3, breaking down vitamin A into a form we can absorb, and maintaining bile acid production and sulfate in the gut. These enzymes are vital to digestion and absorption of nutrients from our food, especially the essential minerals zinc and magnesium, which are often low in our diets to begin with. Glyphosate has been shown to literally draw out essential minerals such as iron, cobalt, and copper and deplete the amino acids tryptophan, tyrosine, and methionine, which are also common deficiencies in patients with celiac disease. Even reproductive issues associated with celiac disease, such as infertility, miscarriages, and birth defects, can be explained by glyphosate.

Many research studies have convincingly shown how glyphosates and other herbicides destroy beneficial gut bacteria and have contributed to the rise in celiac and other autoimmune diseases in the past fifty years, including the obesity and autism epidemics, infertility, depression, Parkinson's disease, Alzheimer's disease, and cancer.[13, 14] In a 2015 report published by the International Agency for Research on Cancer (IARC), the World Health Organization identified glyphosate as a probable human carcinogen.[15] Several countries in the European Union have banned this herbicide as a result. Studies being performed on human urine and blood in the European Union, where use of GMO wheat is drastically lower and even banned in many countries, are raising concerns about the safety of using this herbicide on human food.[16] Yet there have been virtually no studies undertaken in the United States to assess glyphosate levels in human blood or urine—even with all the new research emerging on the microbiome.

Traditional bakeries in France and other countries throughout Europe historically have adhered to use of only certified non-GMO wheat flour that is grown, harvested, and milled in the European Union to avoid cross-contamination with U.S.-grown GMO wheat flour. This adherence to locally sourced ingredients is just one of the many long-held secrets of the infamous French baguette. Unfortunately, today it is increasingly difficult to find organic, non-GMO wheat flour, even in French bakeries. French millers are now importing less expensive U.S. wheat into France and milling it into flour. It has become difficult to know whether even flour imported from countries like France is U.S.-grown GMO wheat or not. According to the Association Française Des Intolérants au Gluten (AFDIAG), France now has the same rate of people who are gluten-sensitive as most other countries.

Probiotic treatments with *bifidobacteria* in conjunction with a gluten-free diet have been shown to relieve symptoms associated with celiac disease, reducing inflammation associated with the affected imbalanced microbiota of celiac patients. Not coincidentally, studies show the same reduction in inflammation can be achieved for those with only a sensitivity to wheat.[17, 18] Luckily, restaurants with gluten-free options are all the rage, and health food stores with gluten-free products have become the norm in most cities. The lacto-fermentation of organically grown wheat also has the potential to reduce gluten levels drastically as well as lessen gluten toxicity. One study that used a culture of sourdough *lactobaccili* and fungal proteases as a sourdough starter found their bread produced a particular strain of *lactobacilli* that lowered gluten levels to 12 parts per million (ppm), a significant reduction from their non-sourdough bread, which had gluten levels of 75,000 ppm.[19] According to gluten-free standards, any product with less than 20 ppm can be labeled as gluten-free, rendering this type of sourdough bread certified gluten-free. Perhaps even more powerful than the lower gluten level is having the lactic acid enzymes necessary for efficient digestion of the wheat plant within the bread itself. Not all sourdough bread is the same, however. Non-sourdough bread made with the same wheat, but without lacto-fermentation, has significantly higher gluten levels.

SUGAR DETOX PHASE II: REFINED GRAINS

After cutting down the grams of sugar in my diet to ten grams a day, I was better able to weed out the cravings coming from my pathogenic flora and began to gain confidence in how to respond to different cues coming from my body. I realized that my sugar cravings usually meant my body needed one of three things—none of which were to consume sugar! Minor short-term sugar cravings that only lasted two to five minutes meant I was looking to sugar as a stimulant and instead needed to rest and activate my parasympathetic nervous system's relaxation response through mindful activity. Stronger, more consistent sugar cravings meant the craving was coming from the pathogenic flora overgrowth that needed to be addressed with diet and herbs. Finally, hunger and sugar cravings too soon after eating meant two things: My blood sugar was out of whack *and* I was probably vitamin and mineral deficient, which meant I wasn't absorbing all the nutrients from my diet. This last one required me to replace all refined grains in my diet with more nutrient-rich whole grains, vegetables, legumes, and healthy fats to keep me satiated in the short-term while I took probiotics and prebiotics to strengthen my gut lining and beneficial flora so I could absorb my nutrients more efficiently and boost my internal nutrient reserves.

During this phase of your sugar detox, I challenge you to clean your cupboards of refined grains, especially wheat products, and find substitutes. It's up to you whether you remove some or all wheat or refined grain products if you suspect they may be causing an inflammatory response in your body.

FIND THE GRAIN EXERCISE

Now I'm going to ask you to look closely at your diet to find out which types of processed grains you consume and how often. Do you consume them once a day, a couple of times a day, or with every meal? Grab your weeklong food journal from chapter 1 and circle the foods that contain unbleached, enriched, or wheat flour. Then count how many times in a week you ate each type of food. To help in this effort, I've included a list of the most common highly processed or refined high-glycemic foods below.

Common Processed Grains to Avoid during Phase II

Check the ingredient list on the items in your pantry. Anything where the first ingredient is unbleached or enriched flour contains a highly processed form of wheat that both spikes our blood sugar and is more difficult for the body to utilize than whole foods. This ingredient is usually the first item for most of the snack foods found in the aisles of modern grocery stores. Examples include:

Bread
Instant oatmeal
Pasta, noodles
Bagels
Pretzels
Tortillas (unless 100 percent stone-ground corn)
Most cereals (except for unsweetened, 100 percent whole grain cereals in
    which you can see the whole grain, such as unsweetened muesli, rolled
    oats, or unsweetened puffed grain cereals).
Granola bars
Graham crackers
Crackers
Dough, piecrust
Muffins
Cookies
Croutons

GERMINATE YOUR GRAINS

Organic whole grains such as brown rice, bulgur wheat, quinoa, amaranth, barley, kamut, spelt, and buckwheat are chock-full of fiber, minerals, and vitamins. A single seed contains all the nutrients to bring a new plant to life, but many of them lie dormant, waiting for water to enter and awaken the nutritious substances sleeping within. Soaking your grains before cooking them allows the grains to get a jump start on the fermentation process prior to reaching your intestines, and helps the tiny seeds begin to germinate and release all these hidden vitamins and minerals more readily, aiding in easier digestion and absorption once they reach your small intestine. Soaking grains, seeds, nuts, and legumes also can help ease indigestion. Germinating, through soaking in water, deactivates phytic acid, which is found in the coating of many seeds and grains, including rice, and binds with minerals, blocking their absorption into the bloodstream. The phytic acid in brown rice, for example, can bind to zinc, magnesium, iron, and copper, pulling these minerals out of your body. Humans do not produce enough phytase, the enzyme required to break down phytic acid. However, the probiotic *lactobacillus* and other bacteria that live in your large intestine can produce phytase—just another reason why having probiotics as part of your everyday diet can prevent nutrient deficiencies and improve digestion. Soaking your rice for at least twenty minutes will begin to deactivate the harmful effects of this acid. Short-grain brown rice, rich in vitamins B5 and B6, is one of my personal favorites. I like to soak it for six to twelve hours before cooking, giving it a plumper, juicier texture and shortening the cooking time to be similar to white rice, about twenty minutes. Cooking brown rice is simple, just add one and a half cups of water to each cup of rice with a pinch of salt and let simmer until all the water is gone—about forty minutes for unsoaked rice.

Whole grain buckwheat is another one of my favorite side dishes. Buckwheat can be soaked for up to twelve hours, but if you're in a hurry you can soak for just twenty minutes and then boil it like pasta and serve with butter and salt. Buckwheat is a quick and easy germinated complement to any meal. When soaking grains, seeds, nuts, and legumes for longer than three to four hours, just be sure to rinse and strain them with fresh cold water every four to six hours.

Soaking your grains and seeds long enough for them to sprout will give you the full nutritional and flora-promoting benefits. Check out the chart in this chapter for time and sprout length to watch for when sprouting. Chickpeas and mung beans, for example, will start to sprout little shoots after three to four days of soaking. Larger, more hearty grains like brown rice, kamut, barley, and spelt can soak for days. If the temperature is right (roughly 75 degrees Fahrenheit), all these grains will start to grow sprout shoots after two to three days. Toss them on top of a salad for a crunchy topping.

Soaking nuts and seeds also makes them easier to digest and allows for the release of nutrients. You will even notice a creamier flavor when snacking on plumped-up soaked almonds, for example. Almonds soaked for six hours develop a rich, creamy, fuller taste and are a delicious snack by themselves, blended into a smoothie, or used to make homemade almond milk. To make homemade nut milk, simply soak a cup of your favorite nuts for two to six hours, then blend in a blender with three parts added water and maybe a pinch of maple syrup or raw honey. Strain with cheesecloth or a fine-mesh strainer and you have delicious, creamy milk you can add to your coffee, smoothie, or

Table 7.1. Soaking and Germination Chart

Nut/Seed	Dry Amount	Soak Time	Sprout Time	Sprout Length	Yield
Almonds	3 cups	8–12 hours	1–3 days	1/8 inch	4 cups
Amaranth	1 cup	3–5 hours	1–3 days	1/4 inch	4 cups
Barley	1 cup	6 hours	12–24 hours	1/4 inch	2 cups
Buckwheat	1 cup	6 hours	1–2 days	1/8–1/2 inch	2 cups
Cashews	3 cups	2–3 hours			4 cups
Flax seeds	1 cup	6 hours			2 cups
Garbanzo beans (chickpeas)	1 cup	12–48 hours	2–4 days	1/2–1 inch	3–4 cups
Lentils	3/4 cup	8 hours	2–3 days	1/2–1 inch	4 cups
Millet	1 cup	5 hours	12 hours	1/16 inch	3 cups
Mung beans	1/3 cup	8 hours	4–5 days	1/4–3 inches	4 cups
Oats, whole, hulled	1 cup	8 hours	1–2 days	1/8 inch	1 cup
Pinto beans	1 cup	12 hours	3–4 days	1/2–1 inch	3–4 cups
Pumpkin seeds	1 cup	6 hours	1–2 days	1/8 inch	2 cups
Quinoa	1 cup	3–4 hours	2–3 days	1/2 inch	3 cups
Spelt	1 cup	6 hours	1–2 days	1/4 inch	3 cups
Sunflower seeds	1 cup	6–8 hours	1 day	1/4 inch	2 cups
Walnuts	3 cups	4 hours			4 cups
Wild rice and brown rice	1 cup	12 hours	2–3 days	rice splits	3 cups

cereal. If you're really hankering for something sweet, throw a Medjool date and a little of your favorite nut butter into the blender for a creamy smoothie.

Low-Glycemic Non-GMO Grains and Wheat Alternatives

Please note: This is not a list of gluten-free grains. Some of these grains may contain gluten.

Almond flour
Chickpea flour
Coconut flour
Whole oats (non-instant), including oat flour
Spelt, including spelt flour
Sprouted organic whole wheat breads
Farro
Kamut
Barley
Brown rice (short grain, long grain), including brown rice flour
Quinoa
Whole buckwheat, including buckwheat flour
Amaranth
Millet
Teff

TAKEAWAYS

- Foods high on the glycemic index contain sugar molecules that can easily be pulled apart and cause a blood sugar spike.
- Refined carbohydrates are higher on the glycemic index than most other foods, sitting right below refined sugar on the glycemic scale.
- High-glycemic foods such as fruit, bread, and cereals can lead to a blood sugar imbalance similar to added sugars, especially when eaten in large amounts or without sufficient fat, protein, or fiber.
- The wheat we consume today has been genetically modified, hybridized, and treated with various chemicals, such as glyphosate herbicides. All of these changes have been shown to disrupt gut flora and cause a number of health conditions.
- Wheat often triggers an immune response that causes inflammation in the intestine and throughout the body, inhibiting the small intestine's ability to absorb and digest nutrients as well as compromising the intestinal wall.

· 8 ·

Sugar Incognito

SUGAR DETOX PHASE III

$\mathcal{N}$ow that we've covered our first and second masked musketeers—processed sugar and refined wheat, the third and fourth masked musketeers are the trickiest of all. One has been hiding behind a "healthy" veil because of its proclaimed calcium content—that's right, I'm talking about milk. In this third phase of your sugar detox, you will learn how to distinguish between dairy products that support your gut health and dairy that sabotages your internal ecosystem.

Several decades ago, in the early 1990s, the U.S. population was advised to cut much of the fat out of their diet, mostly by eating low-fat dairy products, and to ramp up carbohydrates by eating more refined grain products. This advice was taught in nutrition classes, printed in Food and Drug Administration (FDA) reports and brochures, touted by the American Diabetes Association (ADA), and promoted nationwide. We were then advised to consult the Food Guide Pyramid designed by the U.S. Department of Agriculture (USDA), which showed images of wheat grains and cereals in the bottom, largest portion of the pyramid, as part of the FDA's recommendation that we increase our carbohydrate intake to replace high-fat dairy products in our diet. At the time this advice was being dispensed, the FDA leadership board was largely composed of former CEOs from some of the largest food industry companies—go figure![1] The FDA was also being heavily lobbied by the dairy and processed food industries trying to sell their refined, packaged food products like cereal and skim milk. Not much has changed since then, unfortunately. The low-fat, high-carb diet promoted in the 1990s is arguably the most harmful nutrition myth of all time, and significantly ramped up the rate of diabetes and obesity, which was already on the rise. Since then, many extensive, long-term longitudinal studies, such as the Women's Health Initiative—the largest nutrition study in history—have shown that there are no health benefits to eating a low-fat diet or consuming a large amount of carbohydrates, and that this type of diet actually can increase the risk of many chronic diseases. Due to both their poor track record of recommendations and the strong relationships that still exist between food industry giants and the FDA and USDA, the USDA My Plate recommendations have lost a lot of their credibility among nutritionists and health coaches worldwide.

I too used to eat a fruit-flavored low-fat yogurt every day and praise myself for eating a high-protein, low-fat food. As it turns out, low-fat dairy products actually contain a disproportionate amount of the monosaccharide (sugar) lactose. Lactose is a disaccharide composed of galactose and glucose, which means milk is also very high in galactose, one of only three monosaccharide sugars that exist in our diet. A cup of skim milk can have ten to fifteen grams of lactose sugar; a cup of plain low-fat yogurt can have nine grams of lactose sugar, which is in addition to any added sugar or fruit sugar that comes in yogurt. Liquid carbohydrates, such as milk, also have an added danger to blood sugar levels. The University of Illinois Extension found that liquid carbohydrates cause a much faster spike of blood sugar than solid carbohydrates such as pasta or bread. They glide right through the digestive tract and into the bloodstream, creating another reason why we might crave these drinks if our blood sugar is out of balance.

THE FATTIER, THE BETTER

All the evidence pointing to high-fat dairy products may come as a shock, given our nation's touting of low-fat dairy products. However, more and more research is confirming that fat, as opposed to the sugar or protein, is indeed the most nutritious ingredient in dairy products, promoting weight loss and reducing the risk of metabolic syndrome. Milk in low-fat yogurt, cheese, frozen yogurt, and other products is stripped of its fat, leaving the sugar lactose and proteins such as whey. Lactose raises blood sugar when the enzyme lactase splits up into the monosaccharides glucose and galactose. Herein lies the controversy over whether milk is a high-glycemic or a low-glycemic food. Because this split takes longer than, say, white bread or table sugar to separate the glucose compounds, some nutritionists still deem low-fat dairy a healthy option for those struggling with blood sugar imbalance or sugar cravings—even recommending low-fat dairy for diabetics. But these nutritionists are overlooking another major factor, that is, the impact dairy has on insulin.

The primary way conventional milk plays with our blood sugar is in disrupting our insulin levels by overstimulating insulin secretion to a much higher degree than can be explained by the lactose sugar content alone. Cream and butter, however, do not have the same effect on insulin levels, and I'll explain why. Insulin is a key player in stabilizing our blood sugar when it gets too high for too long. It is also vital in shuttling nutrients into our cells. One study in the *European Journal of Clinical Nutrition* (2005) found that when participants switched to dairy as their primary source of protein for just seven days, their blood-insulin levels doubled. There were even signs of insulin resistance just one week into the high-dairy diet. Research at Dartmouth Medical School shows that milk, much like sugary and high-glycemic foods, creates prolonged elevations of insulin that stimulate androgen receptors in the body and can give rise to insulin resistance.[2] However, there is still something else at play here. Research studies in Sweden and Denmark suggest that milk, more than other sugary foods, has both short-term and long-term effects on insulin and therefore blood sugar regulation due to the amino acid composition of the dairy proteins in milk—specifically the amino acids leucine, valine, lysine, and isoleucine, which are insulin-stimulating proteins. These proteins are largely found in whey, which explains why whey protein elicited the biggest insulin response in these studies.[3] There is also evidence that skim milk in particular has been found to produce more insulin resistance than whole milk, due to higher amounts of lactose and whey and lower levels of milk fat. Aside from imbalanced blood sugar control, higher insulin levels also open up our inflammatory pathways, leading to inflammatory conditions such as seasonal allergies, skin conditions, weight gain, migraines, arthritis, and chronic pain.[4,5] Researchers have found that the consumption of dairy and high-glycemic foods both lead to increased insulin levels, which particularly exacerbate the development of acne.[6,7]

There has not yet been comprehensive research looking at whether fresh, whole, unpasteurized milk has the same impact on insulin levels. However, it would be interesting to compare, and judging from the results of skim versus whole milk, it is likely that raw whole milk would have a much lower impact on insulin levels than either conventional milk product due to its high fat content and the presence of enzymes and probiotics to help digest the proteins and sugars found in milk more efficiently.

I'll never forget Susie's story. Susie suffered from severe allergies and had exhausted all treatments traditional Western medicine had to offer when she came for her first appointment with Dr. Wise while I was working at her office. Susie had tried antihistamines, decongestants, steroid nasal sprays, allergy shots, eye drops—you name it. Instead of walking out with yet another prescription, Dr. Wise decided to run some tests to find out if Susie had any food allergies that might be weakening her immune system. Her main clue was that Susie also had symptoms indicating inflammation in her digestive tract. As it turned out, Susie had a minor dairy allergy that was both weakening her immune system and triggering her body's inflammatory response through increased mucus in her respiratory tract and throughout her intestines. Once she stopped eating dairy, her allergy symptoms disappeared altogether—as long as she continued to avoid dairy.

The way many food allergies play out in our body begins in the digestive tract and the interplay with the microflora that resides there—specifically the small intestine, where the largest portion of our microbiome lives. If we lack the enzymes or beneficial flora necessary to digest a specific food properly, or if the food has been refined and processed in a way that has removed the helpful bacteria and enzymes that aid in digestion, as is the case with conventional milk products, an inflammatory reaction in our gut can develop. If all the proteins are not broken down properly into their amino acids, small clumps of partially undigested proteins will remain. Then, if the gut lining of microflora has been weakened for any of the numerous reasons we've discussed, those tiny particles can easily pass through our gut wall and find their way into the lymphatic system. There they will be identified by the body's security guards, our immune cells, which cannot recognize them in their partially undigested form, and they will be attacked as if they are a toxic foreign substance, even though they are just tiny bits of food! Every time our immune cells encounter that same particle, they will issue the same inflammatory response, and be more seasoned and well prepared to attack it. Our system's reaction can thus become more and more severe as this process continues over the years.

PASTEURIZED MILK AND DIGESTION

Although we've been drinking milk for centuries, the liquid we consume today is very different than it was in the past. Less than one hundred years ago milk was always consumed raw, fresh, and whole fat due to its short shelf life in an era before refrigerators. Milk was not heated with our modern-day pasteurization process designed specifically to kill all microbes found in milk. This meant milk contained all the fats, enzymes, and microorganisms—including probiotics—our bodies needed to fully digest and absorb all its nutrients. In fact, it's the probiotics in unpasteurized milk that secrete the enzyme lactase, which our bodies need to break down lactose, likely the cause for so many milk and dairy allergies these days. Unpasteurized milk retains all its healthy fats and beneficial microflora, both of which allow our digestive system to metabolize it efficiently. Many of the vitamins and minerals found in milk, including calcium, cannot be absorbed by our bodies without fat, enzymes, vitamin D, and probiotic bacteria present. Many of these vitamins and minerals are also removed in today's pasteurized, refined version. The presence of these protective, nutritious parts of raw milk wards off any significant blood sugar spikes and supports our immune system, digestion, and microbiome by adding vital probiotics to our digestive tract. Looking back, it makes perfect sense why milk became a staple part of our diet over millennia. It was chock-full of vitamins and probiotics, an ideal source of food for our microbiome! However, the hyper-processed milk we drink these days, transported hundreds of miles after high-heat pasteurization and filtration, no longer has any of these health benefits—making it almost obsolete as a source of high-quality nutrition.

Even calcium in milk is poorly absorbed without phosphatase and vitamin D present. The first, an essential enzyme for metabolizing calcium, is killed during the pasteurization process, and the latter, vitamin D, abundant in raw cream, is filtered out and removed from conventional milk. The absence of these two key elements means we are not even absorbing the majority of the calcium and arguably many other vitamins found in pasteurized, refined milk! Current research suggests vitamin D may be more important than calcium in protecting our bones, due to its role in metabolizing calcium and other protective functions.[8] One large longitudinal population-wide study where 100,000 men and women were followed for twenty years found that high milk intake was actually associated with higher mortality and a higher rate of hip fractures in women.[9] Three glasses of milk a day was associated with nearly twice the risk of premature death! There are countless studies showing that consumption of conventional dairy products during childhood does not promote bone mineralization.[10]

The notion of skim milk products being health-conscious foods is arguably one of the most overstated notions in nutritional medicine. In fact, the highest risks of bone fractures occur in nations with the highest consumption of dairy. In countries with the lowest consumption of milk products, such as Japan, the rates of osteoporosis and hip fracture are the lowest. Why is this the case? In addition to lots of fish and seafood, green tea, sesame, and minimally processed grains, elements of the Japanese diet include loads of green leafy vegetables in addition to fermented, probiotic-rich soy, miso, and pickled vegetables. Green leafy and other colorful vegetables are some of the highest sources of calcium and other minerals in our modern diet. Combining these sources of calcium and minerals with fermented products not only improves our digestion and absorption of these minerals, but also bolsters our microbiome and overall metabolism. This aspect of their diet awards the Japanese their strong bones and visibly well-known healthy disposition.

Don't be too quick to put all dairy on your blacklist though! Despite milk and low-fat dairy's effect on insulin, it's not all bad. Whole-fat dairy products such as organic butter and organic whole-fat yogurt actually have nutritional benefits that are often overlooked. Aside from the fact that the majority of nutrients naturally found in milk are the fat-soluble vitamins A, D, E, and K, which require fat to be present for the body to absorb them from our food, whole milk (used to make yogurt) also contains essential fatty acids such as linoleic and linolenic acid, which are only found in milk fat. Some studies have actually found milk fat to be protective against type 2 diabetes. A study published in the December 2010 issue of *Annals of Internal Medicine* followed 3,736 men for ten years and found that those who had the highest blood levels of fatty acids from whole-fat dairy foods had 60 percent less chance of developing type 2 diabetes than men with the lowest blood levels of fatty acids from dairy products. Another study that looked at the consumption of all various forms of dairy products and the connection to diabetes risk found only yogurt intake to be protective against type 2 diabetes.[11] Total dairy consumption was not found to be protective.

Much like wheat, the majority of the milk from cows in the United States is subsidized by the government. Farmers are incentivized to produce a higher quantity of milk, as they are paid by the gallon, rather than quality milk led by market demand. The use of hormones, a diet consisting of refined corn and wheat, and antibiotics to fight the infections that these added hormones and unhealthy diet result in, are all used to increase milk production at the expense of creating a highly nutritious product. While the average cow produced 5,300 pounds of milk per year in 1950, today the average cow produces more than 20,000 pounds per year.[12] Our increased consumption of these cheap, non-organic, subsidized milk products have further led to many of the nutritional deficiencies and chronic illnesses that abound today. Recombinant bovine growth hormone (rBGH), the main hormone used in dairy production, increases milk production by increasing levels of another hormone known as insulin-like growth factor (IGF-1). rBGH is a man-made hormone that's been banned in the European Union, Canada, and other countries due to research linking this hormone with the development of breast, colorectal, prostate, and other cancers.[13] According to *Science News*, 80 percent of all U.S. feedlot cattle on conventional farms are injected with hormones.[14]

When choosing your dairy products, try to find organic and high-fat dairy whenever possible. (See Table 8.1.) Organic farms feed their cows organic food (hay, silage, and grains), and the cows must receive at least 30

Table 8.1. **Dairy List**

Organic Dairy Farms	Dairy Produced Without rBGH
Alta Dena Organics	Alta Dena
Butterworks Farm	Ben & Jerry's Ice Cream
Harmony Hills Dairy	Breyers Ice Cream*
Horizon Organic	Brown Cow Farm
Morningland Dairy	Crowley Cheese of Vermont
Natural by Nature	Dannon
Organic Valley Dairy	Franklin County Cheese
Radiance Dairy	Grafton Village Cheese
Safeway Organic Brand	Great Hill Dairy
Seven Stars Farm	Lifetime Dairy
Straus Family Creamery	Stonyfield Farms
Stonyfield Organic	Yoplait
Wisconsin Organics	

percent of their food intake from pasture during the growing season, which is about 120 days of the year. Organic farms are required to use organic fertilizers and pesticides in addition to avoiding antibiotics. If a cow becomes ill and needs to be treated with antibiotics, she may never be milked in an organic herd again and must be removed from the farm. The result is that organic farms produce 43 percent less milk per day than conventional farms, but arguably with significantly higher amounts of nutritious vitamins and minerals from being pasture-fed part of the year and without harmful hormones and antibiotics that destroy our microflora. Organic dairy products generally cost a bit more than conventional, but as you can see it's a worthwhile investment.

What the conventional dairy industry doesn't tell us, amid all their marketing on how we need milk to build strong bones, is that calcium is naturally found abundantly in many, many other foods such as white beans, salmon, leafy greens, almonds, and oranges. Most milk substitutes (coconut milk, almond milk, rice milk, hazelnut milk, cashew milk) also fortify their milks with calcium, although we don't absorb added vitamins and minerals nearly as well. A small amount is naturally found in both almond milk and rice milk. You can get calcium a variety of ways in whole foods, and especially in a vegan whole foods diet that includes organic fermented vegetables, miso, tempeh, and small amounts of tofu.

After removing added sugar and refined wheat from my diet, I further removed the low-fat dairy foods I ate most often and searched for milk-free or high-fat diary substitutes. Personally, I found I actually preferred the taste of sugar-free almond milk, coconut milk, and other nut-based dairy alternatives to regular milk. For example, Califia almond milk is made from organic almonds and is by far the most creamy substitute for whole milk. Coconut milk creamers taste amazing in coffee or lattes and imitate dairy cream with their similar thick, smooth texture. I kept organic yogurt as a staple in my diet but replaced low-fat yogurt loaded with sugar-sweetened fruit with plain, high-fat yogurts that contain lots of healthy bacteria (such as *Lactobacillus acidophilus*, also called *L. acidophilus*, *Bifidobacterium bifidum*, and *Streptococcus thermophilus*).

There are also a few good almond milk yogurts on the market these days, such as Kite Hill (avoid the added sugar varieties), which also makes delicious vegan cream cheese. I've found that adding a little honey-sweetened straw-berries or fresh blueberries is so much tastier than the too-sweet fruit jelly I used to scrape up from the bottom of the container. My favorite way to have yogurt is to slice a handful of strawberries and drizzle a tiny bit of maple syrup (half a teaspoon) on top, letting them sit and soften for a few minutes until they become sweet. Adding just a tiny bit of syrup or raw honey enhances the natural sweet juices in the strawberries, and the end result is delicious. Making just a few small changes like this can not only reduce your overall sugar intake without compromising your sweet tooth, but will also provide you with more vitamins and nutrients by switching to foods that are naturally sweet superfoods. This will help you stabilize blood sugar and reduce sugar cravings without sacrificing sweet foods altogether while keeping under your allotted ten grams a day.

In summary, when choosing dairy products, choose organic butter, whole-fat (aged) cheeses, and yogurts that contain added enzymes and probiotics to help with digestion, being careful to watch out for "added sugar" in the ingredient list. Remember that five to ten of the grams of sugar listed on the nutrition label are the sugars naturally found in dairy, in addition to any remaining added sugars. Check the list of ingredients on the package to make sure enzyme cultures and probiotics such as *lactobacillus* are included. Large amounts of dairy will have a negative impact on insulin and androgen levels, so it's smart to avoid dairy if you are prone to acne or have unstable blood sugar. If you are lucky enough to have clear skin, there are proven benefits to including a small amount of whole-fat butter, aged cheese, and dairy-based yogurt in your diet! Otherwise, stick to nut milk and coconut varieties.

You're probably starting to worry that the only way to be free of sugar habits and to heal your body is to completely stop eating all of these foods—no cream in my coffee, no wine with dinner, no bread! Well, you can breathe a sigh of relief, because you don't need to cut these foods out entirely. What's most important is to begin to limit the quantity of these foods in your diet and increase the relative percentage of whole, plant-based foods and foods high in fat and fiber. Unless you are a body builder or pregnant (building a baby), your body really doesn't require much protein to maintain health. Check out the list of alternatives and some suggested brands below to find delicious substitutes for milk or other dairy products.

GUIDE TO RETHINKING DAIRY IN YOUR DIET

Here's an exercise to help you think about the dairy in your diet. Brainstorm through your daily eating routine and make a list of all the dairy products in your diet.

Circle or highlight all the ones that are high in fat *and* contain beneficial enzymes or probiotics—these are totally safe to remain in your diet.

Cross out all the ones that are low in fat *or* contain processed sugars—it's best to avoid these altogether.

The rest (not circled or crossed out) are okay to have in your diet, but *at a minimum*.

Here's a sample list of dairy products to help jump-start this exercise:

Original List

- milk
- high-fat organic cream
- regular low-fat regular cheese
- hard aged cheese (containing enzymes)
- regular low-fat vanilla sweetened yogurt
- high-fat yogurt containing probiotics
- ice cream
- Parmesan cheese, feta cheese, goat cheese
- high-fat regular cream cheese
- cream or cheese-filled pastries

Revised List

- ~~milk~~
- high-fat organic cream (reduced but not eliminated)
- ~~regular low-fat regular cheese~~
- **hard aged cheese (containing enzymes)**
- ~~regular low-fat vanilla sweetened yogurt~~
- **high-fat yogurt containing probiotics**

- ~~ice cream~~
- **Parmesan cheese, feta cheese, goat cheese**
- high-fat organic cream cheese (reduced but not eliminated)
- ~~cream or cheese-filled pastries~~

HEALTHY REPLACEMENTS

For the items you crossed out or are trying to reduce, substitute:

- **Non-Dairy Milks/Creams:** organic almond milk, coconut milk, hazelnut milk, hemp seed milk (there are so many to choose from these days!), coconut creamer, organic soy creamer. If you are looking for a dairy alternative, be careful, 94 percent of soy is genetically modified and therefore relies heavily on large amounts of pesticides, herbicides, and other chemicals to grow. If you're going to buy anything with soy, make sure it's organic.
- **Yogurts:** organic whole milk yogurt containing beneficial probiotics, organic cultured almond, cashew, or coconut yogurt.
- **Cheeses:** aged hard cheeses containing enzymes such as fresh Parmesan, feta cheese in moderation, cultured organic almond or cashew cheese such Kite Hill cashew cream cheese, or my personal favorite, Miyoko's Creamery, which makes creamy vegan cheeses using cultured organic cashews and cultured vegan butter using organic coconut oil and organic cashews.
- **Desserts:** low-sugar coconut and cashew milk ice cream, almond milk ice cream, frozen banana and fruit smoothies. Check out So Delicious Dairy Free products, which have a variety of coconut milk and cashew milk ice cream flavors to choose from. Be cautious of the sugar content in these.

WHAT'S THE DEAL WITH ALCOHOL?

Milk is not the only liquid carbohydrate to watch out for. For most forms of alcohol, even though most of the sugar has been consumed by bacteria and yeast during the fermentation process, these beverages are still liquid carbohydrates that spike our blood sugar more than solid carbohydrates—especially in the case of mixed drinks, which also contain added sugars. Beer and wine in particular disrupt blood sugar and foster *Candida* and other sugar-loving microbes due to the high content of yeast and refined liquid carbohydrates. But it's the residual effect on our blood sugar after drinking that may be more worrisome. Hours after drinking a glass of wine, for example, our body enters a hypoglycemic state, which stimulates sugar and fat cravings. The liver plays an important part in blood glucose regulation by steadily releasing glucose into the blood throughout the day, but alcohol sabotages our liver's ability to release glucose into the blood. This condition causes a blood sugar drop, sugar cravings, a hypoglycemic state, and can lead to insulin resistance.[15] Alcohol also inhibits ghrelin secretion—a chemical that communicates to our brain that we are full. As you can see, there are a number of reasons why you might find yourself starving and overly tired the morning after a night out drinking.[16] The next day your body's blood sugar levels are out of whack, and to readjust, your body goes into desperate hunger mode. The resulting imbalanced blood sugar level may last anywhere from a few hours to days or a week, based on your own predisposition to blood sugar imbalances. Beer and wine also adds more yeast to the body when we are trying to create an environment uninhabitable for pathogenic yeast and fungi—such as *Candida*—to live.

Not all that long ago, alcohol was always consumed fermented, unpasteurized, and unfiltered, which preserved the enzymes and B vitamins for our bodies—plus, it contained a whole bunch of healthy flora for our gut. If you've ever had kombucha, you know how energized, rather than tired, you feel after drinking one of these raw, unpasteurized, fermented drinks—not to mention the reduced time spent on the toilet. Humans used to get all these health benefits from consuming wine and beer! Now all we get from pasteurized, processed alcohol is a blood sugar spike, especially when it's consumed on an empty stomach.

The effects of alcohol on blood sugar, and especially hypoglycemia, makes drinking more dangerous for those with diabetes. Alcohol can also make hypoglycemia medications less effective. You've probably been told to *never drink on an empty stomach*. Food helps to slow the rate at which your body digests the alcohol, so that your blood glucose isn't dramatically impacted by all the empty calories found in alcoholic drinks. Drinking a full glass of water for every alcoholic drink consumed will help keep you hydrated and aid your liver in its necessary detox process after drinking. Switching to lower-alcohol drinks will also help keep your blood sugar more balanced.

We've long known that alcohol poses a burden on the liver, but only now are we starting to understand why, and it too starts in the gut. Recent scientific evidence suggests that alcohol itself, when devoid of any beneficial microbes, can alter the delicate equilibrium in our intestinal environment, leading to gut dysbiosis and leaky gut.[17] When our gut microbes are exposed to alcohol in the intestine, research in both mice and on humans shows a decrease in bacterial diversity over time and changes in composition and abundance of beneficial microbes.[18, 19] This is most likely due to changes in the pH of the colon and disturbances in intestinal absorption of nutrients, including several vitamins, after consuming alcohol.[20] Our healthy gut microbes play an important role in the absorption of minerals and vitamins from our food. However, when there is mucosal damage caused by alcohol and increased permeability of the gut lining, this impedes our body's absorption of calcium, magnesium, folic acid, vitamin B12, thiamine, vitamin B6, and vitamin A, C, D, E, and K absorption.[21] This "leaky gut" also allows bacterial toxins from the gut into our bloodstream, which make their way to our liver, placing an added burden on our liver to cleanse our blood of these toxins in addition to the alcohol we've consumed.[22] As I mentioned earlier, if you suspect you may have an imbalanced gut flora, it's best to stop drinking alcohol until your microbial balance is restored. However, if you don't think *Candida* or other imbalances are a problem for you, then by all means keep a small amount of wine or organic beer in your diet.

Spanish locals are by far the biggest wine lovers I've ever met. Wine is offered at any café or restaurant and often comes with an appetizer at no extra charge. Given this sort of culture, you would think people living in Spain drink a lot of wine, but they actually drink very little. Wine is served to fill only one-eighth of each glass, about one-quarter the serving size of wine in most restaurants in the United States. Even if someone orders two glasses of wine in Spain, they are still drinking half of an average American serving. If you are going to reintroduce wine or other types of alcohol after your sugar detox phase, be careful how much you are drinking and experiment with having smaller amounts. If it would be unthinkable to give up your glass of wine every night, maybe try reducing it to a Spanish-size serving.

An important consideration to make when choosing which alcoholic drinks to keep in your diet is how they are manufactured. Ever wonder why microbrewery and craft beer tastes so good? Most of the widely known and mass-produced beers are pasteurized, but some microbreweries and even some larger breweries skip the pasteurization process, both in the keg and the bottle, offering unpasteurized, unfiltered beer that offers a naturally strong flavor you can't find in pasteurized, filtered beer. Similar to milk, the pasteurization process kills all the beneficial bacteria, enzymes, and other microorganisms that aid in the efficient digestion of fermented alcoholic drinks. The pasteurization process of wine and beer is done primarily to extend the shelf life of these products, at the expense of the quality of the product. Of course, if you buy unpasteurized wine or beer, or make it at home, make sure to keep it in a cold place to prevent spoilage. Like all live foods, unpasteurized beer and cider contains live enzymes—yeasts (full of B vitamins) and healthy bacteria including probiotics, which occur naturally during the fermentation process. However, since most beers are made from fermented wheat, if you think gluten increases inflammatory pathways in your body, it's better to avoid beer and stick to other types of alcohol beverages.

MY SUGAR, DAIRY, AND ALCOHOL DETOX

When I first discovered I needed to take a break from eating sugar and refined grains and drinking alcohol to heal my gut and take care of my health, I felt paralyzed. I had just moved to a completely new side of the country immediately following college and knew no one. I worried how I would meet new people and make friends if I was excluding myself from participating in the timeless rituals of socializing at bars, drinking alcohol, or eating pizza. In my fearful-mind's eye I caught a glimpse of myself alone in my kitchen on a Saturday night wearing my pajamas and baking gluten-free, sugar-free muffins, babbling on and on to an entourage of cats surrounding me. Even the thought of taking a break from alcohol or wheat for a few short months seemed social suicide for a young person in a new town, far away from familiarity.

Rather than giving in to my fears and isolating myself, I decided to go to the bars and concerts and parties anyway, and simply not drink or eat anything I would regret. Eventually I realized I could still participate in all the same activities I did before, but without sugar, refined grains, or alcohol. I taught myself how to prepare my own snacks ahead of time when going to social events, in case there wasn't much I could eat there. The first time I went to a party knowing I wasn't going to drink any alcohol, I was extremely nervous. *What will people say or do if they realize I'm not drinking*, I worried. As the night went on, I laughed away my anxiety as I came to the realization that as long as I had some kind of drink in my hand, everyone either just assumed there was alcohol in it or they simply didn't care what I was drinking! I started to have a lot of fun pretending to be tipsy and laughing a little too loud along with everyone else in the room. I also realized that any friends who I feared wouldn't understand my choice not to drink, or who might judge me or think less of me just because I wasn't drinking alcohol, were not the sort of people I wanted to surround myself with.

Gradually, I overcame my limiting beliefs that I needed to be eating and drinking like everyone around me to have fun, meet people, or be social. I came to experience the benefits of self-care with every single thing I put in my mouth—after all, I was the one who would need to face this choice the next day when I felt tired, sick, or bloated. Every choice I made that aligned with my inner values of taking care of my body bolstered my integrity and made me feel more like the creator of my life, undisturbed by outside influence. This new confidence in myself turned out to be way more attractive to potential new friends than trying to "fit in."

Over time, it became clear which foods were making me sick and which foods were making me feel whole and energetic. The less I consumed of poor-quality foods, the more my energy levels and social life soared. I had a lot more stamina—which helped a lot at late night dance parties. Additionally, my new-found clear mind from not drinking alcohol actually helped me have more mean-ingful, quality exchanges with new and old friends—ultimately improving all my relationships. The worst outcome I feared when I first started avoiding sugar and alcohol, that it would lead to social isolation and loneliness, soon proved to be dead wrong. Avoiding sugar and alcohol turned out to be the antidote, not the cause, for all my social anxieties at the time. I was soon shocked and pleased to discover I had more high-quality, meaningful friendships than ever before.

DAIRY-FREE RECIPES

Coconut Milk Chai Smoothie

Ingredients:

> ½ cup whole raw cashews
> ¼ cup So Delicious Coconut Creamer, or another brand of coconut cream
> 1 frozen (previously ripe) banana
> 1 teaspoon Chai Spice mix (cardamom, anise, ginger, cloves, cinnamon)
> 4 ice cubes
> Maple syrup (optional)

Directions:
Soak whole raw cashews in water for 1 to 2 hours. Blend with remaining ingredients until smooth. Add 1 teaspoon maple syrup for added sweetness. Makes 1 serving.

Decaf Coconut Milk Frappe

Ingredients:

> ¼ cup So Delicious Coconut Creamer, or another brand of coconut cream

1–2 shots of organic decaf espresso or ½ cup strongly brewed French
   press decaf coffee
4 ice cubes
2 tablespoons raw honey or raw coconut sugar

Directions:
Blend all ingredients until smooth. Makes 1 to 2 servings.

Berry Fruity Smoothie

Ingredients:

1 frozen banana
1 cup frozen or fresh★ strawberries, raspberries, and/or blueberries
1 tablespoon maple syrup
4–6 tablespoons store-bought cultured nut yogurt
⅛ cup water or nut milk
★Add 4 large ice cubes if berries are not frozen

Directions:
Blend all ingredients until smooth. Makes 1 to 2 servings.

TAKEAWAYS:

- Milk contains an abundance of lactose, one of the three main disaccharides in our diet next to sucrose and maltose.
- Milk and other low-fat dairy products have been found to stimulate insulin more than most foods. This effect on insulin can lead to insulin resistance, the precursor to hypoglycemia and type 2 diabetes.
- Keep dairy products to a minimum. However, including a small amount of organic high-fat cheese, butter, or yogurt with added enzymes and probiotics can be beneficial for your blood sugar and intestinal tract.
- Alcohol is also a liquid carbohydrate and should be avoided during your sugar detox phase. After this phase, introducing small amounts is fine, as long as you are not trying to get rid of *Candida*.

· 9 ·

Balanced Bellies

$\mathcal{N}$ow that you've likely started to make a few changes to your diet to put a halt to any sugar frenzy in your gut, it's time to continue building up your healthy flora and increasing the biodiversity of your microbiome. What do those little guys need to grow? What types of foods should you eat during and after your sugar detox to make sure you're repopulating your inner garden with the right fertilizer? How do you create the right internal soil? How do you plant new strains of healthy bacteria? In this chapter we will go over specific foods, plants, teas, and activities that, when incorporated into your routine, will help your beneficial belly microbes flourish and begin to establish an enhanced, new and improved microbiome.

When you think about microflora and rebalancing gut bacteria, likely probiotic supplements are the first thing that comes to mind. Green powders that combine probiotics with prebiotic food, such as Green Vibrance and VitaMineral green drinks, are the ideal all-in-one seed plus fertilizer probiotic supplement for your new micro-garden. These green drink powders contain a variety of probiotic strains along with all the super-nutrient foods they need to eat to flourish. If you are trying a new green drink and having trouble acclimating to the flavor, try adding a little juice to the water/powder mix to make it more palatable.

Thinking back to our hunting-gathering days, we often relied on wild greens, herbs, wild mushrooms, and other medicinal plants to sustain us during times when fresh meat or fish were hard to come by. This is where we got many of the healthy microbes our bodies needed and that we evolved to become dependent on over millennia—vegetables and wild herbs don't run away, after all. Compared to hundreds of thousands of years of living as foragers, our modern world—which has only been around for a blink of an eye in human history—doesn't provide us with the nutrients our gut biome has come to rely on. Unless you have your own medicinal herb garden and regularly incorporate these plants into your diet, green superfood drinks, which combine dozens of these vital foods into one, have become a modern-day necessity for many.

If it's difficult to consume raw fermented foods or a prebiotics-rich green drink on a consistent basis at first, a slightly less effective alternative is to take a daily probiotic supplement. This is an easy, convenient way to help repopulate the gut with beneficial strains that support our health and reduce unfavorable bugs. They are easy to take with you to work or while traveling. Probiotic supplements also have the ability to remodel the microbiome of an individual recovering from antibiotics treatment.[1] When choosing a probiotic supplement, you may need to try a couple of different kinds before you find the right one for you. Be sure to switch to a new formula every 6 months to help diversify your microflora.

When you start a new probiotic or green drink, it's common to experience temporary symptoms such as gas, bloating, and looser stools. These are all signs that healthy bacteria are recolonizing your gut. You also may notice a difference in the frequency of bowel movements, especially if you usually only go once a day or less. When taken consistently for a month you may notice an improvement in your mood, digestion, and energy levels and possibly even a reduction in cravings for carbohydrates when taking your probiotic daily. Your appetite may even increase slightly, with cravings for plant-based foods and high-quality fats rather than sugary snacks. These healthy cravings are a sign that your metabolism is operating more efficiently as a result of adding probiotics. I recommend taking a green drink or probiotic capsule with at least six to ten different strains of beneficial flora. Remember, we're trying to increase diversity, so the more the better. The key probiotic strains to look for in your supplement are *Lactobacillus acidophilus*, *Bifidobacterium bifidum*, and *Saccharomyces boulardii*. Some new innovative companies are even offering a sequencing-based clinical microbiome screening test that looks for beneficial and pathogenic microorganisms associated with specific infections, digestive problems, and weight gain and recommends a unique probiotic blend for you. Beneficial strains to look for when purchasing a probiotic supplement that is suited to your specific health needs are *Bifidobacterium bifidum*, *Bifidobacterium longum*, *Bifidobacterium breve*, *Bifidobacterium infantis*, *Lactobacillus acidophilus*, *Lactobacillus bulgaricus*, *Lactobacillus brevis*, *Lactobacillus casei*, *Lactobacillus rhamnosus*, and *Saccharomyces boulardii*.

FLORA FOOD

While a probiotic green drink or supplement may be the easiest thing to start doing and is always one of my first recommendations to my health coaching clients, it really only is a ripple in the surface of the ocean of possibilities when it comes to bolstering your internal flora. There's a whole world of various prebiotic and probiotic foods that can not only improve your digestion and immune function, but also add exciting new flavors to every single meal. Ever wonder what they meant in your high school biology class when they said human cells cannot digest fiber? Digesting fiber is the job of our flora, and healthy flora need a specific type of fiber-rich carbohydrate to flourish. It may sound shocking to hear "Eat more fiber-rich carbohydrates" given the popularity of low-carbohydrate diets these days. And hold on a second, didn't I just go over all the reasons carbohydrates are bad because they spike our blood sugar? Let's make a crucial distinction here, between refined carbohydrates, the kind you find in packaged foods and soft drinks, and whole-seed grain and legume carbohydrates like brown rice, quinoa, black beans, and lentil or split pea soup. Whole grain-, vegetable-, and legume-based carbohydrates contain specific forms of fiber that serve as the ideal food for our beneficial flora to live off of. They play a vital role in populating the gut with healthy microbes.[2, 3]

The reason low-carb diets are so successful for losing weight and reversing chronic illnesses and inflammation comes from the replacement of refined grain flours and sugar with fiber-filled fruits and vegetables—not the elimination of fiber-rich whole grains like millet, brown rice, amaranth, and buckwheat or legumes like lentils and edamame. Quite honestly, any diet that removes sugar and refined white flour is going to improve our weight, energy, and immune function, just as any diet that adds prebiotic-rich plants is going to boost our microbiome and result in greater health. Some of the foods that contain the highest amount of readily available dietary fiber for our microbiota are in fact *high-carbohydrate foods* like buckwheat, split peas, oatmeal, and lentils. Note that whole grains don't contain quite as high a concentration of vitamins, minerals, enzymes, and beneficial bacteria as vegetables and herbs, so if you are concerned you may be vitamin or mineral deficient, then it can be helpful to reduce the amount of whole grains in your diet while you build back your internal nutrient stores through more nutritionally dense plant foods.

When I was in college, both traveling and studying other cultures during my anthropology undergraduate years, I noticed that most of the poorest communities around the world weren't struggling with the epidemic of metabolic and autoimmune problems we suffer from in the United States. I didn't think it just a coincidence, even then, that they all incorporated various whole, non-refined grains in their diets as staple foods in lieu of bread. While spending time in northern and southern Africa, I noticed many communities used stone-ground millet to make everything from bread to breakfast cereal. Even in well-off Western countries like France, you won't find convenience stores stocked with rows of sweets and refined wheat products like we have in the United States. Instead, you'll see small, local corner stores in every neighborhood stocked with dried lentils and beans, fresh fruits and vegetables, a variety of grain staples like rice, barley, and buckwheat, grass-fed antibiotic-free cheeses and meats from local farms, and only a small selection of snack foods like crackers or fresh-baked breads to go with the cheeses. There is a noticeable absence of the candy, soda, and processed sugar and wheat products that you see in the United States. In fact, the original Parisian Creperie didn't serve refined white flour crepes; the crepes were made of 100 percent buckwheat flour and thus gluten-free! If you venture away from the main streets serving white, sugary crepes to unsuspecting tourists and turn down the old cobblestone alleyways, you can still find some of these traditional creperies today, serving steaming, buttery buckwheat crepes filled with local aged cheese—rather than Nutella—to the locals, who know the secret to a delicious, nutritious microbial feast full of healthy fiber and fats.

Foods with the highest fiber content include artichokes, lima beans, peas, edamame, brussels sprouts, raspberries, blackberries, avocados, pears, and barley, to name a few. When vegetables, whole grains, and healthy fats (fat helps us absorb many of the essential vitamins and minerals in our food) become the focus of each meal, as in the example of the original Parisian buckwheat crepe, your gut will be happier, your liver livelier, and your immune system will perform like a finely tuned instrument. Foods naturally high in fiber also slow the amount of time it takes for any processed, refined grains that may still be lurking in your diet to be digested, thus curbing the rate at which glucose enters the blood and helping to stabilize blood sugar, in addition to providing soluble fiber to the intestines that supports the growth of healthy gut flora. Healthy fats like avocados, nuts, seeds, and coconut, sunflower, flaxseed, and walnut oils also help to mellow blood sugar spikes, as well as aid in absorption of vitamins and minerals from our food and curb our appetite by increasing satiety after meals.

Nearly all fresh vegetables and fruits are good sources of fiber. However, there are a number of super-microbial foods that are high in both insoluble and soluble fiber, such as flaxseeds, brussels sprouts, asparagus, collard greens, broccoli, eggplant, summer and winter squash, turnips, rutabagas, parsnips, and beets. Fruits high in soluble fiber such as bananas, apricots, grapefruit, mangoes, and oranges are delicious blended into a fruit smoothie or a green smoothie with spinach or kale. Eat as many bushels of brightly colored vegetables as your heart desires, including artichokes, peas, asparagus, bean sprouts, bell peppers, celery, cucumber, fennel, mushrooms, okra, onions, string beans, summer squash, tomatoes, and zucchini, making sure to include starchy veggies like organic potatoes and yams, which your gut flora especially love.

Fiber supplements are all the rage and can be helpful with constipation, but they do not contain fermentable fibers that our microbiota can break down. Non-fermentable fiber supplements like these allow our stool to absorb more water and result in an easier bowel movement; however, they are not contributing to our microbiota's health or diversifying the species of healthy flora. The more fermentable fiber you consume, the more diverse your microbiota. If you eat a lot of onions, you will gain more inulin-fermenter microbes. If you eat apples, you will accumulate pectin-fermenting microbes. Mushrooms will help the mannan-eating microbes populate your gut. Every organic plant you consume contains a diverse subset of microbes that break down and digest carbohydrates, ready to take up residence in your gut, decrease inflammation, and bolster your immune system. The variety of plants in your diet serves as one of the main methods to change and maintain the diversity in your gut.

Dietary fiber and starches act as precursors to the fermentation process that creates short-chain fatty acids such as acetate, propionate, and butyrate. Many short-chain fatty acids have been found to reduce the risk of developing gastrointestinal disorders, cancer, and cardiovascular disease. Butyrate, for example, nourishes the colonic mucus, which helps us absorb nutrients from our food and protect us from developing leaky gut syndrome leading to inflammation.[4] Butyrate is produced in the gut after consuming foods like barley, oats, brown rice, bran, and herbal tea. Butyrate has also been shown to improve our brain health as well, preventing neurodegeneration and promoting regeneration of brain cells.[5] We've already gone over how the gut microbiota and nervous system interact in the gut-brain axis, producing neurotransmitters such as GABA and serotonin, and regulating the immune system. It has also been shown that some microbe-derived metabolites, such as butyrate, upon entering our blood circulation, can cross the blood-brain barrier to produce neurotransmitters, alter epigenetic markers, and produce metabolites that help generate increased energy (ATP) from our food.[6]

Similar to fiber, polyphenols are not completely absorbed from the gastrointestinal tract. They are also metabolized by gut flora, which causes them to behave like a prebiotic-type substance. Polyphenols are found in coffee, vegetables, tea, and even wine. Studies examining the polyphenols found in teas, however, are at the top of the list. Numerous studies have found that the beneficial flora of subjects who consume green, black, and herbal teas flourish due to a diet rich in polyphenols.[7, 8] The polyphenols found in black and green tea have been found to promote healthy gut bacteria and reduce inflammation. Herbal teas, including ginseng tea, have been found to have prebiotic-like effects on gut microbiota similar to black or green tea, in addition to aiding in creation of the butyrate-producing bacteria so crucial to gut health. Studies at the Center for Cancer & Inflammation Research in China found that the herbal tea saponins found abundantly in ginseng tea promote butyrate production, in addition to enhancing *bifidobacterium* and *lactobacillus,* in mice.[9, 10]

A current popular diet that focuses on feeding our beneficial flora is the macrobiotic diet. This diet originated in Japan as a diet to cure illness, and is the diet that Madonna so famously has followed throughout her successful career as a dancer, singer, and songwriter. Ever wonder what her secret is—how a woman over fifty seems to retain her youth so easily? Her personal chef, Mayumi Nishimura, has helped not only Madonna retain the radiance and beauty of her youth, but countless other celebrities including Sting, Brad Pitt, Gwyneth Paltrow, Stella McCartney, and Guy Ritchie. The secret to looking and feeling young, even as we age, is to keep our microbiome rich with a garden of macrobiotic foods that feed beneficial flora, including starchy roots such as ginger and yams, whole grains and legumes, loads of steamed, stir-fried, and sautéed vegetables, small amounts of meat, fish, traditional green and herbal teas, and, of course, raw fermented foods like kimchi, sauerkraut, pickled vegetables, miso, and tempeh.

ADDING FERMENTED FOODS TO YOUR DAILY DIET

Aside from feeding your beneficial bacteria and flora with probiotic supplements and prebiotic plant foods, you can also increase the diversity of the microbes in your gut by eating raw fermented foods like organic yogurt, raw cheese, kefir, coconut kefir, miso, apple cider vinegar, sauerkraut, kimchi, raw pickled vegetables including pickles and pickled ginger, sourdough ancient grains, unpasteurized wine and beer, and kombucha. Properties of fermented foods make these foods protective against disease and cancer, lower our cholesterol, regulate our immune system, balance our blood sugar, and ward off pathogenic microbes and inflammation with their antimicrobial and anti-inflammatory properties—all while adding probiotics and other beneficial microbes.[11] As long as it is organic and raw (unpasteurized), fermented food is bound to have a high quantity of healthy living flora to help repopulate your gut and rebalance your microbiome.

The process of fermentation is completely natural and easy to effect because beneficial bacteria live on the surface of all living plants, fruits, and vegetables. *Lactobacillus,* for example, is the primary probiotic bacteria living on the surface of cabbage and the reason its fermented version, sauerkraut, is so high in this particular beneficial bacteria. When you make sauerkraut, you simply put shredded cabbage, water, and salt in a glass mason jar with a cloth draped over the top and leave it in a cool, dark cabinet for three to ten days while the *lactobacillus* and other probiotics work their magic. The *lactobacillus* bacteria feed off the natural sugars found inside the cabbage and turn into lactic acid. Enzyme by-products like lactic acid found in sauerkraut and other pickled vegetables act as a preservative so that they don't spoil quickly. These fermented foods can be kept in the fridge for three to six months.

The fermentation process does many incredible things aside from preservation. It also helps us absorb the nutrients in our food and adds up to twenty times the amount of vitamin C compared to regular cabbage. Fermentation also adds vitamins like B2 (riboflavin), B9 (folate), B12, and vitamin K.[12] We always make sure to have a batch of homemade sauerkraut in our fridge at home and often add a couple of forkfuls to our plate at most meals. Our two-year-old daughter also likes to munch on it occasionally and often asks for some when she sees us eating it. Kimchi, made from Chinese cabbage, carrots, red pepper flakes, chili peppers, and sometimes ginger and garlic, is a bit too spicy for our daughter's taste buds, but many people love the serious spiciness of this popular South Korean condiment. Eating fermented kimchi on a daily basis has been shown to lower total glucose, total cholesterol, and LDL ("bad cholesterol") after just one week.[13]

Another reason for the rise in lactose intolerance and food allergies lately is a result of the hyper-processing and additives used in foods today to prevent spoilage. The same foods that used to be the most healing and healthful for our gut, such as jarred soups and vegetables, pickles, and fermented dairy, are now ridden with pesticides and chemical preservatives. Additionally, the pasteurization of dairy products kills off all the beneficial enzymes and bacteria we need to digest them. The salt added to fermented vegetables such as sauerkraut and kimchi acts as a natural preservative so there is no need for pasteurization and other additives.

Although kefir, like yogurt, is made from pasteurized milk, dozens of different strains of probiotics are added back in for the fermentation process. This makes kefir one of the most microbe-rich foods available, with ten to thirty different strains of beneficial flora in a single serving. Because of the high density of probiotics breaking down the lactose sugars, kefir is also completely safe for those who are lactose intolerant.[14] All dairy products available prior to refrigeration and pasteurization used to involve some sort of fermentation involving bacteria breaking down and digesting the sugars while giving us a healthy dose of probiotics—the ideal food for our gut!

Yogurt is the next best thing to kefir at the modern supermarket or farmer's market. Be sure the brand of yogurt you buy lists the probiotics on the back, and look for probiotic names such as *lactobacillus* and *bifidobacterium*. Raw cheese is the easiest unpasteurized dairy product to find these days in most major supermarkets. Raw cheese from grass-fed cows, sheep, or goats often includes *thermophillus*, *bifidus*, *bulgaricus*, and *acidophilus*.[15] When shopping for dairy in today's market, search for organic dairy products made from grass-fed cows or, even better, goats or sheep, so you are not getting products laced with antibiotic and GMO corn from conventional grain-fed dairy farms.

For those of you who can't eat much dairy, like me, there are many alternatives available today including coconut kefir, almond milk yogurt, and cashew-fermented cheeses (my personal favorite). These products contain the same probiotic strains found in dairy-based products, albeit in slightly lesser amounts.

One of my favorite fermented foods to eat is miso. You can add miso to almost anything to enrich the flavor of your food. I mix a tiny amount with peanut butter and spread it on whole grain crackers and apples, or use it as a sauce for pasta with a little added water and oil. Made from fermented soybeans, rice, or barley, miso soup is the most popular way to eat miso and is served in Japanese restaurants. Miso is a staple food in Japan, often eaten at breakfast to stimulate the digestive system and energize the body for the day. Shio koji, similar to miso but in liquid form, is used as a seasoning ingredient with fish, meat, and vegetables. It looks like a rice porridge and is slightly sweet. Depending on the length of fermentation and amount of water, it can come in puree, paste, or solid form.

Kombucha, a fizzy, cider-like drink made from fermented black tea, has become a new fad in the United States and is now sold in most supermarkets and even corner stores and pharmacies right next to fruit juices and soda. Remnants of the murky mass of bacteria known as the "mother" lurking in the bottle may be off-putting, but this culture is actually the life-giving source of probiotics that gives this drink its warranted health properties. Kombucha is loaded with beneficial bacteria, amino acids, B vitamins, and enzymes that improve digestion, energy, and liver detoxification. Kombucha is by far the easiest fermented food to make in your own kitchen and will save you a ton of money. All you need is a live scoby or "mother," as they are called, which can be ordered online or borrowed from a friend, and a half cup of leftover raw store-bought kombucha to get started. If you know anyone who makes kombucha frequently, they will happily hand over a "kombucha baby," a new layer on the mother, which is the result of every batch of kombucha they make and just requires a little help to be separated from its mother. This "kombucha baby" can now serve as your new "mother." Here are the directions for making your own kombucha at home:

1. To make one quart of kombucha, boil 4 cups of filtered water, free of chlorine or fluoride, in a pot on the stove.
2. Wait for the water to come close to a boil, then add ⅓ cup organic white sugar and two black tea bags (or 2 teaspoons of loose tea). Stir

until the sugar dissolves. The water should be hot enough to steep the tea but does not have to be boiling.

3. Turn off the stove and let the tea steep while the water cools to 68–85°F. You may remove the tea after 10 to 15 minutes, or leave it until cool for a stronger kombucha tea.
4. Remove tea bags and pour tea into a glass jar. Add ½ cup kombucha from store-bought or a previous batch of homemade kombucha and the active scoby "mother" into the jar with the brewed tea.
5. Cover the jar with a thin cotton kitchen hand towel or a coffee filter and secure with a rubber band.
6. Allow the mixture to sit undisturbed at 68–85°F, out of direct sunlight, for four to twenty days, or to taste.

Note: The longer the kombucha ferments, the less sugary it will be and the more vinegary it will taste. I like to wait until it is no longer sweet and then add a little fruit juice for flavor when I serve it. When your kombucha is done, save the scoby and enough liquid from the bottom of the jar as your starter tea for the next batch.

FLAVOR-RICH FLORA FOOD

When I lived in Eugene, Oregon, the local natural foods market became my hunting grounds for new flora-friendly foods. I didn't have much money to spend, so I frequented the bulk food aisles regularly and filled dozens of tiny plastic baggies with new flavor agents with high hopes they would satisfy my desire for flavor and tantalize my taste buds in place of milk, sugar, and refined flour in my diet. Fresh and dried herbs, spices, and tea are all chock-full of antioxidants and phytochemicals metabolized by the gut microbiota as another ideal source of energy.[16, 17] I'd fill up each plastic pocket with just a couple of tablespoons of spices and herbs like Zen green tea, ground-up marjoram, crispy ginger, sandy garlic powder, salty garlic powders, grassy rosemary, savory oregano, cinnamon sticks, bark-colored anise and cloves, and aromatic cardamom pods. I also experimented with small samples of different grains and legumes like short-grain brown rice, French blue lentils, and Indian orange lentils. The Indian diet opened up a new frontier for me, namely coconut oil, coconut milk, and a variety of spices including turmeric, cumin, curry, and coriander. From cooking many Ayurvedic recipes, I learned that sautéing fresh-chopped garlic, onions, and ginger added flavor to nearly any savory dish I was cooking. Sautéed ginger and garlic in a stir-fry are also the perfect antidote for an overgrowth of bacteria or fungi. Garlic is a natural antifungal and antimicrobial, and ginger, a powerful prebiotic and ideal flora food, has been proven highly effective at reducing inflammation and supporting the digestive system.[18] Indian food is traditionally served with rice, which made it easy for me to avoid flour and bread. I found a simple coconut milk stir-fry that was easy to make on a weekly basis, with the total cooking time under thirty minutes. It's warm, comforting, and satisfying, especially in the cooler months. The best part is leftovers the next day, which always seem to taste even better when the spices infuse deeper into the vegetables. You'll find my recipe at the end of the chapter.

When your diet revolves around fresh and fermented vegetables, non-flour whole grains, and healthy fats at every meal, your blood sugar will stabilize and you'll avoid the elevated insulin levels that lead to inflammation. Add a small amount of hormone- and antibiotic-free chicken or beef to a vegetable dish for a savory flavor enhancer and just the right amount of fat, but be cautious when purchasing your meat and know where it comes from. Remember how dangerous antibiotics are for our gut flora? Most conventionally raised meats and livestock are routinely treated with antibiotics from birth, and in fact, 80 percent of the antibiotics sold in the United States are used in meat and poultry production.[19] The reason we are at risk when we consume these products is due to the presence of antibiotic-resistant superbugs present in meat and poultry, which can transmit to us when we consume them.[20] This is why so many health organizations, including the American Medical Association, American Public Health Association, Infectious Disease Society of America, and the World Health Organization have all issued statements calling for a reduction in the use of antibiotics for animal food production. Choose organic, hormone- and antibiotic-free sources of meat, fish, and seafood whenever possible to protect your gut flora balance. Some healthy choices for meats and seafood include wild salmon, herring, Atlantic mackerel, arctic char, anchovies, sardines, oysters, mussels, trout, and halibut, as well as pasture-raised eggs, chicken, and beef for their omega-3 EPA and DHA. EPA/DHA found in these foods has been shown to reduce inflammation, improve glucose tolerance, and protect against development of pre-diabetes.[21, 22, 23] Avoid large fish like tuna as much as possible due to their high mercury content, overfishing, and farming practices linked to pollution and contamination.

Chromium is essential for blood sugar balance. Increased glucose and insulin levels are the primary signs of chromium deficiency. Making chromium-rich foods a part of your everyday diet will create a long-term habit of supplying your body with bio-friendly nutrients rather than relying on a supplement, which is more difficult to absorb in your intestinal tract compared to whole foods. Oysters and mussels are very high in chromium, and grass-fed beef has been found to have higher levels of chromium and other minerals than conventional meats. Other foods high in chromium include brewer's yeast, broccoli, mushrooms, and to a slightly lesser degree, barley, oats, green beans, tomatoes, romaine lettuce, and potatoes.

FLORA-FRIENDLY PLANT PROTEINS

It's a win-win for our gut and our muscle tone when we turn to local, organic plants and whole, non-refined grains as our primary sources of protein. Contrary to popular belief, it's actually easy to get sufficient protein from plants alone. With the exception of vitamin B12—which is very difficult to get in a vegetarian diet—most other vital nutrients are actually higher in plants than animal products. High-protein diets based in animal protein have been shown to increase the net dietary acid load, which requires our kidneys to filter out the excess acid through our urine.[24] This effect can be tested for with a simple pH strip test.

Another reason to turn to local, organic plants for protein is that plants are the primary source of minerals in our diet. Unfortunately, conventionally grown fruits and vegetables severely lack mineral content compared to organic produce. A study that compared conventionally grown apples, pears, potatoes, wheat, and sweet corn (some of the most heavily sprayed crops) with organic versions found that the organically grown foods were 63 percent higher in calcium, 73 percent higher in iron, 110 percent higher in magnesium, 178 percent higher in molybdenum, 91 percent higher in phosphorus, 125 percent higher in potassium, and 60 percent higher in zinc.[25] Sadly, minerals are becoming more and more scarce in a world where soil depletion and aggressive agricultural methods have literally stripped the minerals and nutrients out of the soil. Magnesium, for example, is a necessary mineral for more than 300 biochemical reactions in the body including maintaining nerve and muscle function, supporting our immune system, hormonal balance, and regulating blood glucose levels. This deficiency of minerals in our soil has translated into conventional produce that is deficient in minerals, and more and more diagnoses of mineral deficiencies by holistic health providers who test for nutritional deficiencies as standard protocol. This outcome is just one more reason why buying local and organic produce is so important. Vegetables high in magnesium such as kale, spinach, and other dark leafy greens, along with avocados, beans, and lentils, are the best way to increase magnesium, hit your daily protein mark, and feed your essential microflora all in one. Nuts, seeds, and fish are also good sources of magnesium. A Harvard University study found that high daily magnesium intake reduced the risk of type 2 diabetes by 33 percent.[26] Magnesium also plays a vital role in our body's use of insulin and regulating blood sugar. Lower intake of magnesium in the diet is associated with increased risk for type 2 diabetes and pre-diabetes. For all these reasons, magnesium is one of the few supplements I take on a regular basis, in addition to eating a whole-foods diet high in leafy greens.

Just as soil needs the right pH and assortment of minerals to grow crops, so does our internal flora. In addition to feeding your healthy flora, eating alkalinizing foods—mineral-rich foods—also provides a stable pH environment in the gut, which the beneficial microflora need to thrive. If you've ever heard of the Alkaline-Acid Diet, you probably wondered why drinking lemon juice, with a pH of 2.0, makes your intestines and urine more alkaline. While lemon juice itself is incredibly acidic due to high citric acid content, what affects the pH of your digestive tract is whether alkaline or acid by-products are produced during the fermentation process that takes place in your intestine. Plants also contain alkaline nutrients such as potassium, magnesium, and calcium, which affect the pH of your gut. When you drink lemon juice, your body quickly metabolizes the citric acid as it enters the stomach, but the mineral content of lemon juice—calcium, magnesium, potassium, copper, and manganese—takes much longer. The minerals need to go all the way through your intestines to be absorbed, with some remnant minerals discharged through the urine.[27] As a result, your urine pH rises. Acidic nutrients such as excessive animal protein and sulfur increase the amount of acid the kidneys must filter out, while alkaline nutrients like calcium and magnesium and potassium ultimately reduce the amount of acid the kidneys need to filter out through urine. Consuming mineral-rich plant foods not only supplies the gut with more desirable microorganisms and provides the ideal food for beneficial flora, but it also helps create the ideal soil pH for the healthy bacteria already there to grow. For all these reasons and more, minerals are more important for our health than ever—perhaps even more than vitamins—and on par with probiotics and prebiotics. Our bodies can't make minerals like they can make hormones and some vitamins. We have to get them from our food. Plants in general are extremely high in minerals. Therefore, all plants will increase the alkalinity of your intestinal flora, and the environment in your intestinal tract will be primed for an abundant biodiversity of microbial flora and fauna.

One cup of dark leafy vegetables like broccoli (seven grams) or spinach (thirteen grams) is adequate protein for one meal. While it can be hard to get vitamin B12 if you are a vegetarian, you can supplement your diet with Bragg Nutritional Yeast or a B12 supplement. I often add a little Bragg Nutritional Yeast to my daughter's brown rice, and she loves it so much she refers to it as her "cheese," requesting I sprinkle more on her brown rice, vegetables, or quinoa pasta. If you have a history of skin conditions and are currently taking a B12 supplement or thinking of taking one, be careful. Potent vitamin B12 supplements may worsen acne[28] and rosacea by interrupting the microbiota of our skin.[29] Natural sources including tempeh, eggs, yogurt, shiitake mushrooms, nori (seaweed), and nutritional yeast are all high in vitamin B12 and good for your skin too. Fish, seafood, and meat are all very high in chromium and B12, and you don't need to eat much to get these necessary nutrients. The China-Oxford-Cornell Study on Dietary, Lifestyle and Disease Mortality found that diets high in whole grains and vegetables prevented chronic illnesses such as obesity, diabetes, and autoimmune disease.[30] Sixty-five rural Chinese counties were compared based on the levels of vegetable consumption, whole grain consumption, and meat and dairy consumption. Researchers found a strong correlation between high animal product consumption (meat and dairy) and autoimmune diseases. This result is likely due to the fact that vegetarian sources of protein like nuts, seeds, and vegetables are chock-full of nutrients and fiber, which feed our beneficial flora, supporting our immune system to help us ward off illness. These are also alkaline foods that make our gut less inhabitable for many types of pathogenic bacteria and disease.[31] Legumes like lentils, chickpeas, and black beans, and whole grains like quinoa and brown rice are high in protein and the perfect fuel for our gut flora. They also happen to be high in iron, another vital mineral we need to get from plants if there is less meat in our diets. Pumpkin seeds, squash, pistachios, sunflower seeds, cashews, and unhulled sesame seeds are all high in iron as well.

REINFORCE YOUR INTESTINAL LINING

A woman named Sharon was struggling with chronic pain, fibromyalgia, and other inflammatory conditions in addition to taking sleep and anxiety medications when she called me to schedule an appointment. She was desperate to try a different approach for her chronic pain and increasing memory and anxiety problems. Her anxiety had reached an all-time high, and her deteriorating health was taking her down a road where she had all but given up hope of ever turning a corner. I explained the important role our gut flora plays in our health and how certain foods, especially refined sugars, wheat, and certain types of dairy can destroy our internal healthy flora, triggering inflammation, anxiety, and sleep disturbances. I also suggested mindfulness exercises, which we started incorporating into our sessions right away. As a way to repair the severe damage in her gut due to her medications and dietary history, I recommended bone broth soup to heal the intestinal lining and support gut microbe health. Immediately she cut out all flora-disrupting foods from her diet and replaced them with homemade chicken and vegetable soup, made with unpasteurized bone broth she bought at her local supermarket. After only seven days on her new diet, her chronic fatigue, inflammation, and chronic pain had drastically improved.

Although she used store-bought bone broth, it can easily be made at home by placing a chicken carcass in a crockpot or large pot, covering in water, and simmering on low heat for eight to twelve hours. You can also use store-bought beef bones for a slightly more savory beef broth. The broth can be used to make a vegetable soup by adding starchy roots, carrots, potatoes, ginger, and onions and hearty leafy greens for protein, such as kale. If you are making chicken bone broth, you can add the chicken meat back in with the vegetables after making the broth for a delicious chicken vegetable soup. Bone broth contains L-Glutamine and an array of vital minerals including calcium, magnesium, potassium, and phosphorus, all of which help repair the gut lining. L-Glutamine can also be bought in supplement form if you don't eat animal products. If you do eat animal products, homemade bone broth contains a highly absorbable form of L-Glutamine. When combined with starchy roots and greens, bone broth soup makes the perfect microbial elixir to help heal your gut microbial garden.

BREAKING THE FAST

Every morning we wake up dehydrated. After an all-night fast without any liquid, the first thing our liver and detox pathways need to wake up and energize is warm water or warm tea. Warm water is more hydrating than cold water because your body doesn't need to adjust the temperature and can absorb it right away.

Your body relies on its natural detox process by way of the liver, lymph system, and intestinal gut flora to break down, attack, isolate, and purge acidic foods, bacteria, viruses, chemicals, and other toxins we consume through our food and are exposed to in our environment. The time you spend sleeping at night is when regular housecleaning for your body kicks into gear. There are four primary toxin removal systems that occur at night: the disposal of cellular waste, the removal of larger waste through your lymph, the processing of toxins by your liver (which go into bile and then the colon for final removal), and the final clearance of waste products through your colon. The hydrating mineral content, enzymes, and alkaline pH of lemon water, for example, makes it a rejuvenating addition to your morning routine and will support your colon with its daily cleansing process. With all the internal cleansing that takes place at night, morning is a prime opportunity to support the continuation of this detox process—since you've already been fasting and cleansing for the past five to eight hours—and the absolute worst time to eat something sugary like refined grain cereal, milk, or other processed foods that deter this natural detox and could even bring it to a halt altogether.

The ideal start to each day is a meal rich in whole fibrous fruits or veggies, unrefined whole grains (oatmeal, granola, buckwheat, grits, millet, etc.), and fermented and probiotic-rich fats such as dairy or a nut-based dairy alternative. Raw honey or monk fruit powder mixed with walnuts or pecans sprinkled on top will add a touch of variety and flavor. Whole grains are not only our flora's favorite food, but also our brain's fuel. Having a meal with whole grains and healthy fats like nuts, eggs, seeds, or yogurt first thing in the morning will help you wake up and get to your to-do list or jump-start your workday. Fresh berries, melons, and citrus fruits also help to hydrate you in the morning. Add either a healthy lean protein (such as almond butter, eggs, protein powder) and a fat (organic butter, avocado, bacon, coconut oil)—for example, avocado on sprouted ancient grain toast with your egg, or almond butter and coconut oil in your oatmeal or granola. Green smoothies, with spinach, kale, fruit, nut butters, and coconut oil added in, are rich in minerals, fiber, and healthy fats and often contain four to six servings of fruits and vegetable in one glass! By supporting your body's daily cleansing process in the morning, you will reap the benefits throughout the day with more energy, a clearer mind, a happier digestive system, and a stronger immune system.

Chickpea Flour Scallion Pancakes with Probiotic Yogurt Topping

Ingredients:

- 1 bunch (about 6–7) scallions, sliced
- 3 tablespoons extra-virgin olive oil, divided
- 2 cups garbanzo bean (chickpea) flour (can also substitute or add a mixture of hazelnut flour, almond flour, and/or coconut flour)
- ½ teaspoon baking powder
- 1 cup whole-fat Greek yogurt
- 1 ½ teaspoons salt
- ⅛ teaspoon pepper
- 2 eggs
- ½ cup almond milk
- 3–4 teaspoons sunflower or coconut oil to cook the pancakes (1–2 teaspoons per batch)

Directions:

1. In a large nonstick skillet, sauté scallions in 1 tablespoon olive oil for 5 minutes, until tender. Set aside.
2. In a large bowl, combine chickpea flour, baking powder, yogurt, salt, pepper, remaining 2 tablespoons olive oil, eggs, and almond milk. Mix until well incorporated, then fold in cooked scallions.
3. Heat 1–2 teaspoons vegetable oil in a nonstick skillet. Pour about 2 tablespoons of batter per pancake and cook at medium heat, 2 to 3 minutes per side.
4. Serve hot with a dollop of Greek yogurt sauce on top. To make the sauce, mix ½ cup whole-fat Greek yogurt with 2 teaspoons freshly squeezed or bottled lemon juice, ⅛ teaspoon salt, 1 teaspoon Dijon mustard, and 2 teaspoons relish or capers.

Yams, Cinnamon, and Honey Breakfast Grain Bowl

Ingredients:

1 cup uncooked brown rice or amaranth
1 large yam
1 teaspoon cinnamon
1 teaspoon nutmeg
½ teaspoon salt
1 teaspoon raw honey
1 tablespoon olive oil (optional for baking yams)
1 tablespoon ghee or organic butter

Directions:

1. Soak uncooked brown rice for at least 6 to 8 hours. It can soak for up to 2 days, just be sure to rinse with fresh water every 4 to 6 hours.
2. After soaking rice, chop a large yam and steam in a pot with water on low heat for 20 to 30 minutes. Or, pour 1 tablespoon olive oil over chopped yams, mix thoroughly, and bake at 400°F for 20 minutes.
3. Rinse the rice, then transfer to a saucepot and add 2 ½ cups fresh water. Add cinnamon, nutmeg, and salt. Simmer on low for 20 minutes.
4. When rice and yams are cooked, scoop rice into a serving bowl, place a handful of cooked yams on top, and drizzle with honey and warmed ghee or butter. Makes 4 servings.

Design Your Own Green Smoothie

I encourage you to try your own smoothie combinations with the ingredients below—get creative! Here's a general format I follow when making a green smoothie:

Base ingredients:

> 1 frozen banana (the riper the sweeter)
> ½ avocado
> ½ cup almond milk
> ½ apple
> 1 cup spinach

Optional ingredients:

> ½–1 cup additional liquid (nut or dairy milk, juice, coconut water, or water)
> Frozen fruit of your choice (such as pineapple or mango) up to the top of the liquid
> A handful of additional greens like kale or spinach
> Protein (nut butters, pea protein powder, sunflower seed butter), 1–2 tablespoons
> 1 tablespoon chia seeds for added antioxidants

THE MOST IMPORTANT MEAL OF THE DAY

I know you've heard otherwise, but *lunch* is really the most important meal of the day. This is the only meal where it's safe to overdo it *a little*, as long as you're eating whole, unrefined, unprocessed foods. It's the time of day your body is actively using all the calories you consume. You require a good-sized, well-balanced meal to fuel your brain and your body for your activities throughout the day. Whether you are crunching numbers all day at the office or running after a little one at home, lunch provides the main fuel you use during that time to perform your best. So choose wisely.

Lunch is the time of day I like to include as much variety as possible to increase satiety and get all the nutrients my body needs. It's very important to include both healthy fats *and* fruits or vegetables, with an optional unprocessed protein like fish, meat, or whole grains. Healthy fats like avocados, olive oil, coconut oil, tahini, pumpkin seeds, sunflower seeds, walnuts, almonds, cashews, and nut butters will increase absorption of fat-soluble vitamins. Avocados are a wonderful lean protein, full of healthy fats, and help meet your daily fiber quota, which feeds your beneficial flora. One avocado provides your body with vitamins A, C, E, K, and B6, along with a huge serving of potassium, all twenty-two essential amino acids, and all eight of the amino acids necessary for the body to form a complete protein. They are easy for your body to digest, and all the protein is usable and readily absorbed by your body due to the high fiber content—ironically, even more protein than steak or chicken, where much of the protein becomes denatured and deranged from cooking.[32] Avocados also contain omega-3 and omega-6 fatty acids, which reduce overall inflammation in the body, aid concentration and memory, and help improve mood.

With that being said, I know how hard it can be to find variety in the middle of the day when you're busy working or running errands. The Spanish have the right idea of taking a siesta in the middle of the day. This allows them to go home and have a full meal with their family, then rest and digest after the meal. Most of us can't do that, of course. For the rest of us, taking a break, even as short as twenty minutes, can improve our digestion, absorption of nutrients, and help manage stress levels. Taking the time to sit down to eat a microbe-balancing and satisfying meal without our computer or any other stressors in front of us gives space to mindfully taste and enjoy our meal.

Steamed Vegetables Over Grains with Ginger-Miso Sauce

Ingredients:

> 1 small butternut squash or 2 delicata squash, sliced into 1-inch cubes
> 1 small bunch broccoli, stalks trimmed
> 2–3 large carrots, sliced thick
> 1 bunch white radishes, trimmed
> 3 tablespoons fresh lemon juice
> 1 tablespoon white miso
> 1 small garlic clove
> 2 teaspoons finely grated ginger
> 1 teaspoon raw honey
> 1 teaspoon toasted sesame oil
> ¼ cup olive oil
> Sea salt and freshly ground black pepper
> Cooked rice or quinoa, for serving

Directions:

1. Fill a large saucepan or pot with 1 inch of water, bring to a boil, and set a bamboo steamer or metal steamer basket inside the pot. Arrange squash across the bottom of the steamer, cover, and cook about 5 minutes. Add broccoli, carrots, and radishes and steam until all vegetables are fork-tender, about 5 to 10 minutes.
2. Meanwhile, blend lemon juice, miso, garlic, ginger, honey, sesame oil, and olive oil in a small food processor or with a handheld immersion blender until smooth. Season with salt and pepper to taste.
3. To serve, place a scoop of rice in a bowl, top with steamed vegetables, and drizzle a generous amount of sauce over the top.

Note: Feel free to swap out vegetables to your liking or what's in season. It is also easy to pack up this meal after cooking to reheat at work or on-the-go.

SUPPER—KEEP IT SMALLER

In our culture, this is the meal where we're most likely to overeat. At the end of the day, our bodies are slowing down, and our digestion is too, which means we may not need to eat very much, especially if it's after 7 p.m. Overeating at dinner is actually the secret to how sumo wrestlers gain a lot of weight quickly. When you eat processed carbohydrates and sugar at the end of the day, at a time when your body isn't active, they are even more likely to be stored as fat. Sumo wrestlers will eat 80 to 90 percent of their calories a few hours before bed, and the result is startling!

Understandably, it's often the only time of day when we have the time to sit and eat a slow, full meal and spend quality time with family and friends. It makes sense why we tend to overeat at this time of the day. However, if you eat dinner after 6:30 p.m., it should really be one of the smallest, lightest meals—similar in size to, or smaller than, breakfast. If the evening is the only time you have to cook a hearty meal, then by all means use that time to cook up a storm. Then, eat a small portion for dinner and pack away a larger portion for yourself for lunch the next day.

Eating slowly, until you are no longer hungry, is one of the most effective ways to prevent overeating and feel more satisfied with less. Make sure to savor every bite and chew your food thoroughly which stimulates salivary enzyme production, to further aid in nutrient absorption. Having lots of colorful vegetables with dinner is a great way to eat less and get lots of fiber which feeds your microbiome. Eating an assortment of vegetables with dinner will fill your belly, bolster your gut flora, and keep your blood sugar steady. In the evening, if I don't have time to prepare a fancy meal, I will often make a simple stir-fry (see recipe below) curry, using onion, ginger, garlic, and dark leafy greens like spinach, Swiss chard, or cabbage—which our beneficial gut bugs absolutely love. Sometimes I'll add in a minimal amount of meat as well.

Spiced Vegetable Coconut Milk Stir-Fry

Ingredients:

> 1 cup brown rice, quinoa, or white rice
> 2 tablespoons coconut or olive oil
> 1 small onion, diced
> 4 cloves garlic, minced (2 tablespoons)
> 2 tablespoons grated fresh ginger (or 2 teaspoons ground)
> ½ cup diced carrots
> ½ cup chopped broccoli florets (and/or green bell pepper, cauliflower, yams)
> Sea salt and black pepper to taste
> 1 tablespoon orange curry powder
> Pinch cayenne (optional for heat)
> 2 (14-ounce) cans organic coconut milk
> 1 cup veggie stock (I use water and bouillon)
> ⅓ cup loosely cut snow peas
> ¼ cup diced tomatoes (or a can of diced tomatoes)

Directions:

1. Begin by rinsing your grain of choice thoroughly in a strainer. Add to a medium saucepan over medium heat with 2 cups water. Bring to a boil, then reduce heat to simmer, cover, and cook for 15 minutes or until the quinoa or rice is light and fluffy. Set aside until serving.
2. In the meantime, heat a large saucepan or pot to medium heat and add 1 tablespoon coconut oil. Add the onion, garlic, ginger, carrot, broccoli, and any other additional veggies you want to throw in. Add a pinch each of salt and pepper and stir. Cook, stirring frequently, until vegetables are softened—about 5 minutes.
3. Add curry powder, cayenne, coconut milk, veggie stock, and another healthy pinch of salt; stir to combine. Bring to a simmer, then reduce heat slightly and continue cooking for 10 to 15 minutes.

4. Add the snow peas and tomatoes in the last 5 minutes so they don't overcook.
5. Taste and adjust seasonings as needed. I usually add another pinch or two of salt.
6. Serve over rice or quinoa, and enjoy!

Organic Tempeh Salad

Ingredients:

3 tablespoons Bragg Liquid Aminos or organic tamari sauce
3 tablespoons olive oil
1 tablespoon nutritional yeast
½ teaspoon garlic powder
Black pepper to taste
1 package (227 grams) organic tempeh
5 cups mesclun greens

Directions:

1. In a large bowl, mix together soy sauce of choice, olive oil, nutritional yeast, garlic powder, and pepper to make the marinade. Cut up one package of organic tempeh into 1-inch-long slices and allow to marinate for 20 to 60 minutes.
2. Grease the bottom of a frying pan with oil, just enough to cover, and place each piece of marinated tempeh into the pan in one layer, evenly spread around the pan. Allow to cook on medium/low heat for 2 to 4 minutes, or until light golden brown. Flip slices of tempeh and cook until the opposite side is golden brown. Remove from heat and let cool on a paper towel.
3. Serve tempeh on top of mesclun greens or lettuce covered with your favorite vinaigrette. You can also add additional toppings such as slices of peppers, shredded carrots, chickpeas, or bean sprouts.

TAKEAWAYS

- Green prebiotic and probiotic drinks and supplements are the easiest, most convenient way to rebalance the gut, help diversify the species of healthy flora, and keep pathogenic strains at bay. Search for a well-researched brand with at least six to ten different strains of beneficial bacteria.

- Fiber-rich whole grain-, vegetable-, or legume-based carbohydrates are the ideal food for both you and your gut flora and should be included in every meal of the day.
- Similar to fiber, polyphenols (found in coffee, vegetables, tea, and even wine) are metabolized by gut flora, which causes them to behave like a prebiotic-type substance.
- Eating fermented foods like yogurt, raw cheese, kefir, coconut kefir, miso, apple cider vinegar, sauerkraut, kimchi, raw pickled vegetables including pickles and pickled ginger, sourdough ancient grains, unpasteurized wine and beer, and kombucha on a daily basis is the best way to keep increasing the diversity of your microbiome and improve your health.

· *10* ·

Tuning In to the Garden Within

You are your own doctor 99.9% of the time.

—Andrew Ahmann, MD,
director of the Harold Schnitzer
Diabetes Health Center at Oregon
Health & Science University

*I*t's time to tune back in to our internal calling. It's amazing how natural it can be to heal our body and discover more clarity when we view our body from the vantage point of an ecological, microbe-abundant community—rather than a machine where we pump in calories and extract energy. Once we wake up to how we have been treating our bodies over many years, we can begin to serve our bodies with the gentle, loving hands of an expert gardener. This is how we can tap into our truest, most innate state and discover that, just like any garden, we need tending to. When we take the time to make our food and life choices from this base reference point, we will begin to make different choices and, as a result, develop a new set of flora that will crave whole foods and relaxation, rather than sugar and stimulants. The state many of us are seeking—an alert, sharp mind and a relaxed, pain-free body—lies in a calm gut and a primordial diet.

The timeless phrase "You are what you eat" has been proven scientifically sound. Our recent understanding of the microbiome sheds light on the fact that the genetic makeup of our bodies seems to be much more changeable than we could have ever imagined. This important discovery gives us the opportunity to change our health for the better with foods that improve the health of our microbiome. When we take a look at the culture we live in, it's really no wonder that our inner micro-garden—which comprises most of the genes in our body and impacts the gene expression of the other 1 percent from our parents—is suffering chronically. We've been disregarding our delicate inner eco-balance with exposure to unyielding stress; a processed, acidic, high-sugar diet; an over-sanitized environment with toxic chemical exposures; and overuse of medications. In doing so, we've damaged our gut barrier and microbiome, leaving us overly vulnerable to harmful bacteria and illness—the very things we were trying to protect ourselves from in the first place.

The odds may be against us, but there are actions we can take every day to protect ourselves from losing essential strains of beneficial flora and to build back a healthy, flourishing inner world of life-giving organisms. Given that sugary foods are so addictive, we require sound evidence and good reason to give up many of our favorite foods. Yet if we can cut down on the foods, medications, and sanitary practices that have been damaging and derailing our inner ecosystem—literally stealing life from within us—we have the chance to rebuild our genetic roadmap from the ground up. This is an opportunity not only to heal ourselves of inflammatory conditions, blood sugar imbalance, and sugar and processed food cravings, but also to move our internal microbial dial toward complete health. Let's be honest with ourselves—is life even worth living without our health?

We've become addicted to being unhealthy, turning to laboratory-made ingredients pretending to be food for our dopamine-derived pleasure, while a whole world is out there calling us back to our roots. As a species, for the majority of our existence we've lived in the outdoors. We prepared all our own foods, lived without access to the processed and refined sugars that now make up 75 percent of our modern diet, and harvested our own crops—all of which provided ample opportunity for exposure to plants and microbe-rich soils. This lifestyle may seem archaic to some, yet it is possible to drastically reduce our exposure to microbe-killing chemicals, even in our modern world, while encouraging restorative micro-exposures to soil-based organisms. Our culture has developed a prejudice against all microbes, without regard to their vital function and without the knowledge that we are composed largely of microbes ourselves. This is why our nation's health is suffering. We must support one another in overcoming discrimination and allow microbes back into our diet and everyday life if we want to restore our collective health. With just a small backyard or a park nearby to frequent, local and organic produce, a variety of raw fermented foods, hormone- and antibiotic-free meats, more time in the kitchen, and less time in the middle aisles of the supermarket, we can re-create our own version of our ancestors' microbe-abundant existence.

Let's not discount the impact our high-speed life is having on our digestion and enteric nervous system, which acts as a hub for 90 percent of the messages sent from our body to our brain. It's time we tuned out all the high-energy, fear-filled monologues on our TVs for foods, medications, information, and stuff we don't need, and reset our priorities around our microbial well-being. These days it seems we are surrounded by voices enticing us to consume products and information that don't support our truest cravings or the microbial friends within us. We don't need to be a famous actor or actress, whose career depends on their looks and health, to prioritize our own health and wellness over everything else. We can choose to do this ourselves every day by adhering to our primitive instincts telling us to get outside, move more, eat sour, fizzy, fermented foods, stay away from packaged food-like substances, and make space in our lives for our minds to settle.

We've long known that fibrous, phytonutrient- and mineral-rich legumes, whole grains, vegetables, herbs, and sea greens protect us from disease and improve our health. Yet only now do we finally understand why. Plants high in phytonutrients and minerals such as magnesium have been proven to reduce inflammation—which in turn reduces pain—encourage muscle relaxation, and improve mood.[1, 2, 3] They also act as prebiotic foods, the ideal food for our gut. Out in the wild, phytonutrients are a plant's main defense against pathogenic germs, fungi, and other threats. These same phytonutrients protect our inner microenvironment from unhealthy microbes, too. As you consume fewer processed foods, increase your consumption of organic fruits and vegetables, and switch to antibiotic-free meats, you are not only retaining microbial diversity that would otherwise be killed off by herbicides and medications found in conventional produce and livestock, but also priming your microenvironment to produce calm-inducing neurotransmitters like GABA and serotonin.

We're moving beyond the now-disproved theory that "a calorie is a calorie." Caloric foods don't have to be a problem or a source of guilt, because all that matters is whether the foods you eat regularly feed the beneficial flora in your gut. A calorie devoid of beneficial microscopic life is most likely only furthering the growth of pathogenic flora and disease and increasing cravings for processed fats and sugar. Eating organic cruciferous and leafy green vegetables such as cabbage, Swiss chard, spinach, and kale helps us retain and build upon our microbial diversity that would otherwise be harmed by pesticides and herbicides in conventional produce. Eating organic dairy and meat free of hormones and antibiotics further protects us from the damaging effect of these medications on our delicate microbiome.

As a nation, we are feeling tired, depressed, and devoid of life, literally because we are eating too many *dead* foods. To experience an increase in energy, stamina, and zest for life, we need to eat *living* foods! When we eat prebiotic fiber-filled whole grains, legumes, vegetables, and herbs and add living microbes through probiotic-rich foods to our diet, we are restocking our favorite microbial friends. Such a diet strengthens our immune system and metabolism, opens detox pathways, and reduces inflammation. In turn, this shift has a huge impact on our mood and our ability to manage stress.

A calorie covered with healthy microbes is solid gold to your metabolism and taste buds—what our gut is really craving. Why do you think fizzy, sour drinks like soda, beer, and wine are so satisfying? The process of fermentation is the original creator of bubbly drinks. For millennia, humans used fermentation to increase shelf life and get nutrients from plant-based foods in the winter. What happened to these rich, pungent, flavorful foods in our diet in the United States? Today, we attempt to re-create these same tastes, textures, and experiences that are most satisfying to us with pasteurization, chemicals, sugar, and food flavorings, when we have no need for many of these modern practices.

It takes courage to live differently from everyone else, and a strong commitment in a world laden with sugar-covered confections and thousands of microbe-killing potions. Even tap water stripped of minerals and full of chlorine is poised to kill living bacteria. Yet there is a way to live without the use of harmful chemicals and overindulgence in processed, sugary foods. In the beginning it may seem like tiny, insignificant changes, yet even I couldn't have imagined how powerful these tiny steps would turn out to be in my own exploration of a new microbe-rich lifestyle.

My journey healing my gut by diversifying the makeup of my gut microbes has been a learning process spanning the last ten years. Starting with first creating an internal environment uninhabitable for pathogenic flora like *Candida* to thrive—by getting rid of sugary foods that contribute to this environment—I then added fermented foods, herbs, teas, and spices to bolster my microbial diversity with probiotic and prebiotic foods.

My first of what would become a regular annual sugar detox for the next decade of my life was only for a few short months many years ago, yet this detox not only transformed my health but set a new course for my life, ultimately inspiring me to get certified as a health coach; introduce fermented foods, medicinal herbs, and essential oil–based personal and home cleaning products into my everyday life; and ultimately write this book. Along the way I've let many external factors get in the way of caring for myself. Ironically, as it turns out, tending to my needs first and getting my own internal ecosystem back into sync not only improves my health and energy levels, but also blossoms my personal relationships and my career path, and, most importantly, allows me to fully enjoy life.

In examining all the groundbreaking research on the microbiome, the amount that we can change our genes and our bodies is dramatic and far beyond what humankind thought was possible just a few years ago. We are only at the beginning of uncovering all the possibilities. Remember the research studies that transposed new microbes into people with dangerously low microbial levels, and how it resulted in not only physical changes—reducing body weight, improving metabolism, and eliminating health conditions—but also changes in personal traits and personality, things we thought unchangeable? It is possible to change the very fabric of "me," and even the perception of a static "me." Now we know the question is not whether it is possible to dramatically transform our health by changing the genetic makeup of our bodies, because we have objective and subjective findings proving it is possible. The question is only *when*. That sugar habit you want to kick, that extra weight you've always wanted to lose, that muscle or joint pain you want to reduce or eliminate, that ever-present anxiety, even that chronic diagnosis you want to address are all fair game. It is not a hopeless trait or state of things. It is about a specific set of microbes that can be changed by tilling your internal soil and adding the right new seeds to the mix—and now you know how to do it. No matter your age, you can take back the reins of your own health. Armed with the knowledge in this book, you now have all the tools necessary to build up your internal immune system.

The impossible is, in fact, possible. So, I pose my last question: "Who do you want to cultivate?"

Notes

INTRODUCTION

1. Sonnenburg, Justin, and Erica Sonnenburg. *The Good Gut: Taking Control of Your Weight, Your Mood, and Your Long-Term Health.* Penguin, 2015, 71.

CHAPTER 1

1. "Glycemic Index and Diabetes."American Diabetes Association. Accessed September 3, 2017, http://www.diabetes.org/food-and-fitness/food/what-can-i-eat/understanding-carbohydrates/glycemic-index-and-diabetes.html?referrer=https://www.google.com/.

2. Menke, Andy, Sarah Casagrande, Linda Geiss, and Catherine C. Cowie. "Prevalence of and trends in diabetes among adults in the United States, 1988–2012." *JAMA* 314, no. 10 (2015): 1021–29.

3. Menke et al., "Prevalence of and trends in diabetes," 1021–29.

4. *National Diabetes Statistics Report, 2017.* CDC. Accessed March 27, 2018, https://www.cdc.gov/diabetes/pdfs/data/statistics/national-diabetes-statistics-report.pdf.

5. Qin, Junjie et al. "A human gut microbial gene catalogue established by metagenomic sequencing." *Nature* 464, no. 7285 (2010): 59–65.

6. Grice, E. A., and J. A. Segre. "The human microbiome: our second genome." *Annual Review of Genomics and Human Genetics* 13 (2012): 151–70. http://doi.org/10.1146/annurev-genom-090711-163814.

7. Hemarajata, Peera, and James Versalovic. "Effects of probiotics on gut microbiota: Mechanisms of intestinal immunomodulation and neuromodulation." *Therapeutic Advances in Gastroenterology* 6, no. 1 (2013): 39–51.

8. Hullar, Meredith AJ, and Benjamin C. Fu. "Diet, the gut microbiome, and epigenetics." *Cancer Journal* 20, no. 3 (2014): 170.

9. Ghosh, Sanjoy, Erin Molcan, Daniella DeCoffe, Chaunbin Dai, and Deanna L. Gibson. "Diets rich in n-6 PUFA induce intestinal microbial dysbiosis in aged mice." *British Journal of Nutrition* 110, no. 3 (2013): 515–23.

10. Ghosh et al., "Diets rich in n-6 PUFA," 515–23.

11. Farias, MM, AM Cuevas, and F. Rodriguez. "Set-point theory and obesity." *Metabolic Syndrome and Related Disorders* 9 (2011): 85–89.

12. Gerard E. Mullin, *The Gut Balance Revolution*. New York: Rodale Inc., 2014, 26–27.

13. Jacobs, Gill, and Joanna Kjaer. *Beat Candida Through Diet: A Complete Dietary Programme for Sufferers of Candidiasis*. Random House, 2012.

14. Bengmark, S. "Nutrition of the critically ill—a 21st century perspective." *Nutrients* 5 (2013):162–207.

15. Mullin, *Gut Balance Revolution*, 26–27.

CHAPTER 2

1. Alcock, Joe, Carlo C. Maley, and C. Aktipis. "Is eating behavior manipulated by the gastrointestinal microbiota? Evolutionary pressures and potential mechanisms." *Bioessays* 36, no. 10 (2014): 940–49.

2. Norris, Vic, Franck Molina, and Andrew T. Gewirtz. "Hypothesis: Bacteria control host appetites." *Journal of Bacteriology* 195, no. 3 (2013): 411–16.

3. Norris, Molina, and Gewirtz, "Hypothesis: Bacteria control host appetites," 411–16.

4. Lyte, Mark. "The microbial organ in the gut as a driver of homeostasis and disease." *Medical Hypotheses* 74, no. 4 (2010): 634–38.

CHAPTER 3

1. Sonnenburg, Justin, and Erica Sonnenburg. *The Good Gut: Taking Control of Your Weight, Your Mood, and Your Long-Term Health*. Penguin, 2015.

2. Ackerman, Jennifer. "The ultimate social network." *Scientific American* 306, no. 6 (2012): 36–43.

3. Frank, Daniel N., and Norman R. Pace. "Gastrointestinal microbiology enters the metagenomics era." *Current Opinion in Gastroenterology* 24, no. 1 (2008): 4–10.

4. Grice, E. A., and Segre, J. A. "The Human Microbiome: Our Second Genome." *Annual Review of Genomics and Human Genetics* 13 (2012): 151–70. http://doi.org/10.1146/annurev-genom-090711-163814.

5. Probiotics Benefits, Foods and Supplements—a Vital Part of Any Diet, http://draxe.com/probiotics-benefits-foods-supplement.

6. Imam, Talha H., MD. "Fungal urinary tract infections." http://www.merckmanuals.com/professional/genitourinary-disorders/urinary-tract-infections-(uti)/fungal-urinary-tract-infections.

7. Ackerman, "The ultimate social network."

8. Urita, Yoshihisa, Motonobu Sugimoto, Kazuo Hike, Naotaka Torii, Yoshinori Kikuchi, Hidenori Kurakata, Eiko Kanda, Masahiko Sasajima, and Kazumasa Miki. "High incidence of fermentation in the digestive tract in patients with reflux oesophagitis." *European Journal of Gastroenterology & Hepatology* 18, no. 5 (2006): 531–35.

9. Chatterjee, Soumya, Sandy Park, Kimberly Low, Yuthana Kong, and Mark Pimentel. "The degree of breath methane production in IBS correlates with the severity of constipation." *American Journal of Gastroenterology* 102, no. 4 (2007): 837.

10. Ackerman, "The ultimate social network."

11. Ackerman, "The ultimate social network."

12. Sender, Ron, Shai Fuchs, and Ron Milo. "Revised estimates for the number of human and bacteria cells in the body." *PLoS Biology* 14, no. 8 (2016): e1002533.

13. Marotz, CA, and A. Zarrinpar. "Treating obesity and metabolic syndrome with fecal microbiota transplantation." *Yale Journal of Biology and Medicine* 89(3) (2016): 383–88.

14. Sonnenburg and Sonnenburg, *The Good Gut*, 71.

15. Ackerman, "The ultimate social network."

16. "Nearly half a million Americans suffered from Clostridium difficile infections in a single year." CDC Newsroom. Accessed March 27, 2018, https://www.cdc.gov/media/releases/2015/p0225-clostridium-difficile.html.

17. Le Chatelier, Emmanuelle, Trine Nielsen, Junjie Qin, Edi Prifti, Falk Hildebrand, Gwen Falony, Mathieu Almeida et al. "Richness of human gut microbiome correlates with metabolic markers." *Nature* 500, no. 7464 (2013): 541–46.

18. Wong, Julia MW, Russell De Souza, Cyril WC Kendall, Azadeh Emam, and David JA Jenkins. "Colonic health: fermentation and short chain fatty acids." *Journal of Clinical Gastroenterology* 40, no. 3 (2006): 235–43.

19. Ghosh, Sanjoy, Erin Molcan, Daniella DeCoffe, Chaunbin Dai, and Deanna L. Gibson. "Diets rich in n-6 PUFA induce intestinal microbial dysbiosis in aged mice." *British Journal of Nutrition* 110, no. 3 (2013): 515–23.

20. Jernberg, Cecilia, Sonja Löfmark, Charlotta Edlund, and Janet K. Jansson. "Long-term ecological impacts of antibiotic administration on the human intestinal microbiota." *ISME Journal* 1, no. 1 (2007): 56.

21. Cotten, C. Michael, Sarah Taylor, Barbara Stoll, Ronald N. Goldberg, Nellie I. Hansen, Pablo J. Sánchez, Namasivayam Ambalavanan, and Daniel K. Benjamin. "Prolonged duration of initial empirical antibiotic treatment is associated with increased rates of necrotizing enterocolitis and death for extremely low birth weight infants." *Pediatrics* 123, no. 1 (2009): 58–66.

22. Bailey, L. Charles, Christopher B. Forrest, Peixin Zhang, Thomas M. Richards, Alice Livshits, and Patricia A. DeRusso. "Association of antibiotics in infancy with early childhood obesity." *JAMA Pediatrics* 168, no. 11 (2014): 1063–69.

23. Turta, Olli, and Samuli Rautava. "Antibiotics, obesity and the link to microbes—what are we doing to our children?" *BMC Medicine* 14, no. 1 (2016): 57.

24. Dethlefsen, Les, and David A. Relman. "Incomplete recovery and individualized responses of the human distal gut microbiota to repeated antibiotic perturbation." *Proceedings of the National Academy of Sciences* 108, Suppl. 1 (2011): 4554–61.

25. Nobile, Clarissa J., and Alexander D. Johnson. "Candida albicans biofilms and human disease." *Annual Review of Microbiology* 69 (2015): 71–92.

26. Jacobs, Gill, and Joanna Kjaer. *Beat Candida Through Diet: A Complete Dietary Programme for Sufferers of Candidiasis.* Ebury Digital, February 29, 2012.

27. Scarpignato, C. "NSAID-induced intestinal damage: Are luminal bacteria the therapeutic target?" *Gut* 57, no. 2 (2008): 145–48.

28. Naglik, JR, SJ Challacombe, and B Hube. "*Candida albicans* secreted aspartyl proteinases in virulence and pathogenesis." *Microbiology and Molecular Biology Reviews* 67(3) (2003): 400–28. doi:10.1128/MMBR.67.3.400-428.2003. http://www.ncbi .nlm.nih.gov/pmc/articles/PMC193873/.

29. Gleason, JE et al. "Candida albicans SOD5 represents the prototype of an unprecedented class of Cu-only superoxide dismutases required for pathogen defense." *Proceedings of the National Academy of Sciences* 111, no. 16 (2014): 5867. http://www .pnas.org.ezproxy.bu.edu/content/111/16/5866.short.

30. Kauffman, Carol A., John F. Fisher, Jack D. Sobel, and Cheryl A. Newman. "Candida urinary tract infections—diagnosis." *Clinical Infectious Diseases* 52, Suppl. 6 (2011): S452–S456. doi: 10.1093/cid/cir111.

31. Rolston, KVI, and GP Bodey. "Fungal Infections." In DW Kufe et al., eds. *Holland-Frei Cancer Medicine*, 6th ed. Hamilton, ON: BC Decker, 2003. http://www .ncbi.nlm.nih.gov/books/NBK13518/.

32. Yemma, J. J., and M. P. Berk. "Chemical and physiological effects of Candida albicans toxin on tissues." *Cytobios* 77, no. 310 (1993): 147–58.

33. Ackerman, "The ultimate social network."

34. "Biologists ID defense mechanism of leading fungal pathogen." *EurekAlert!* Accessed October 21, 2017, http://www.eurekalert.org/pub_releases/2004-06/ru-bid 062504.php.

35. "Biologists ID defense mechanism of leading fungal pathogen." *EurekAlert!*

36. Fan, Di, Laura A. Coughlin, Megan M. Neubauer, Jiwoong Kim, Min Soo Kim, Xiaowei Zhan, Tiffany R. Simms-Waldrip, Yang Xie, Lora V. Hooper, and Andrew Y. Koh. "Activation of HIF-1α and LL-37 by commensal bacteria inhibits *Candida albicans* colonization." *Nature Medicine* 21, no. 7 (2015): 808. doi: 10.1038/nm.3871.

37. Vázquez-González, Denisse, Ana María Perusquía-Ortiz, Max Hundeiker, and Alexandro Bonifaz. "Opportunistic yeast infections: Candidiasis, cryptococcosis, trichosporonosis and geotrichosis." *Journal der Deutschen Dermatologischen Gesellschaft* 11, no. 5 (2013): 381–94; quiz 394. doi: 10.1111/ddg.12097.

38. Jacobs and Kjaer, *Beat Candida Through Diet.*

39. Chedid, Victor, Sameer Dhalla, John O. Clarke, Bani Chander Roland, Kerry B. Dunbar, Joyce Koh, Edmundo Justino, Eric Tomakin RN, and Gerard E. Mullin. "Herbal therapy is equivalent to rifaximin for the treatment of small intestinal bacterial overgrowth." *Global Advances in Health and Medicine* 3, no. 3 (2014): 16–24.

40. Dupont, PF. "Candida albicans, the opportunist. A cellular and molecular perspective." *Journal of the American Podiatric Medical Association* 85, no. 2 (1995): 104–15. http://www.ncbi.nlm.nih.gov/pubmed/7877106.

41. Hostetter, Margaret K. "Handicaps to host defense: Effects of hyperglycemia on C3 and Candida albicans." *Diabetes* 39, no. 3 (1990): 271–75.

42. Odds, F. C., E. G. Evans, M. A. Taylor, and J. K. Wales. "Prevalence of pathogenic yeasts and humoral antibodies to candida in diabetic patients." *Journal of Clinical Pathology* 31, no. 9 (1978): 840–44.

43. "Finding a single mechanism for hypertension, insulin resistance, and immune suppression." UC San Diego Jacobs School of Engineering. Accessed on July 14, 2017, http://jacobsschool.ucsd.edu/news/news_releases/release.sfe?id=744.

44. Axe, Josh. *Eat Dirt: Why Leaky Gut May Be the Root Cause of Your Health Problems and 5 Surprising Steps to Cure it.* HarperCollins Publishers, 2016.

45. David, LA et al. "Diet rapidly and reproducibly alters the human gut microbiome." *Nature* 505 (7484) (2014): 559–63. doi: 10.1038/nature12820.

46. "Are Your Health Problems Yeast Connected?" The Yeast Connection. Accessed on September 15, 2016, http://www.yeastconnection.com.

47. Chedid et al., "Herbal therapy is equivalent to rifaximin for the treatment of small intestinal bacterial overgrowth," 16–24.

CHAPTER 4

1. "How Much Sugar Are Americans Eating," *Forbes* website. Accessed October 24, 2017, http://www.forbes.com/sites/alicegwalton/2012/08/30/how-much-sugar-are-americans-eating-infographic/.

2. "What the World Eats," *National Geographic*. Accessed December 14, 2017, https://www.nationalgeographic.com/what-the-world-eats/.

3. Ahmed, Serge H. "Is sugar as addictive as cocaine?" *Food and Addiction: A Comprehensive Handbook* (2012): 231–37.

4. Lenoir, Magalie, Fuschia Serre, Lauriane Cantin, and Serge H. Ahmed. "Intense sweetness surpasses cocaine reward." *PLoS One* 2, no. 8 (2007): e698.

5. Colantuoni, Carlo, Pedro Rada, Joseph McCarthy, Caroline Patten, Nicole M. Avena, Andrew Chadeayne, and Bartley G. Hoebel. "Evidence that intermittent, excessive sugar intake causes endogenous opioid dependence." *Obesity* 10, no. 6 (2002): 478–88.

6. "Advertising spending of the food and beverage industry in the United States in 2013, by medium (in thousand U.S. dollars)." Statista: The Statistics Portal. Accessed December 14, 2017, https://www.statista.com/statistics/319053/food-beverage-ad-spend-medium/.

7. Rupp, Rebecca. "Surviving the sneaky psychology of supermarkets." The Plate, *National Geographic*. Accessed December 14, 2017, http://theplate.nationalgeographic.com/2015/06/15/surviving-the-sneaky-psychology-of-supermarkets/.

8. Rupp, "Surviving the sneaky psychology of supermarkets."

9. Préstamo, G., A. Pedrazuela, E. Penas, M. A. Lasunción, and G. Arroyo. "Role of buckwheat diet on rats as prebiotic and healthy food." *Nutrition Research* 23, no. 6 (2003): 803–14.

10. Zhou, Albert Lihong, Nancie Hergert, Giovanni Rompato, and Michael Lefevre. "Whole grain oats improve insulin sensitivity and plasma cholesterol profile and

modify gut microbiota composition in C57BL/6J mice–3." *Journal of Nutrition* 145, no. 2 (2014): 222–30.

11. Iſland, J. R., H. G. Preuss, M. T. Marcus, K. M. Rourke, W. C. Taylor, K. Burau, William Solomon Jacobs, W. Kadish, and G. Manso. "Refined food addiction: A classic substance use disorder." *Medical Hypotheses* 72, no. 5 (2009): 518–26.

12. Nesse, Randolph M. "Evolution and Addiction." *Addiction* 97, no. 4 (2002), 470–71.

13. Avena, Nicole M., Pedro Rada, and Bartley G. Hoebel. "Evidence for sugar addiction: Behavioral and neurochemical effects of intermittent, excessive sugar intake." *Neuroscience & Biobehavioral Reviews* 32, no. 1 (2008): 20–39.

14. Lenoir, Serre, Cantin, and Ahmed, "Intense sweetness surpasses cocaine reward."

15. Aeberli, Isabelle, Philipp A. Gerber, Michel Hochuli, Sibylle Kohler, Sarah R. Haile, Ioanna Gouni-Berthold, Heiner K. Berthold, Giatgen A. Spinas, and Kaspar Berneis. "Low to moderate sugar-sweetened beverage consumption impairs glucose and lipid metabolism and promotes inflammation in healthy young men: A randomized controlled trial." *American Journal of Clinical Nutrition* 94, no. 2 (2011): 479–85.

16. Jameel, Faizan, Lisa G. Wood, Manohar L. Garg, and Melinda Phang. "Acute effects of feeding fructose, glucose and sucrose on blood lipid levels and systemic inflammation." *Lipids in Health and Disease* 13, no. 1 (2014): 195.

17. Spreadbury, Ian. "Comparison with ancestral diets suggests dense acellular carbohydrates promote an inflammatory microbiota, and may be the primary dietary cause of leptin resistance and obesity." *Diabetes, Metabolic Syndrome and Obesity: Targets and Therapy* 5 (2012): 175.

18. Kuo, Lydia E., Magdalena Czarnecka, Joanna B. Kitlinska, Jason U. Tilan, Richard Kvetňanský, and Zofia Zukowska. "Chronic stress, combined with a high-fat/high-sugar diet, shifts sympathetic signaling toward neuropeptide Y and leads to obesity and the metabolic syndrome." *Annals of the New York Academy of Sciences* 1148, no. 1 (2008): 232–37.

19. Tietjen, G. E., M. Karmakar, and A. A. Amialchuk. "CRP and migraine in young adults: Results from the ADD health study." In *Headache*, vol. 56, no. 8 (2016): 1397.

20. Konturek, Peter C., T. Brzozowski, and S. J. Konturek. "Stress and the gut: Pathophysiology, clinical consequences, diagnostic approach and treatment options." *Journal of Physiological Pharmacology* 62, no. 6 (2011): 591–99.

21. Konturek, Brzozowski, and Konturek, "Stress and the gut."

22. Aeberli, Gerber, Hochuli, Kohler, Haile, Gouni-Berthold, Berthold, Spinas, and Berneis, "Low to moderate sugar-sweetened beverage consumption."

23. Grün, Felix, and Bruce Blumberg. "Environmental obesogens: Organotins and endocrine disruption via nuclear receptor signaling." *Endocrinology* 147, no. 6 (2006): s50–s55.

24. Martinez-Zaguilan, Raul, Elisabeth A. Seftor, Richard EB Seftor, Yi-Wen Chu, Robert J. Gillies, and Mary JC Hendrix. "Acidic pH enhances the invasive behavior of human melanoma cells." *Clinical & Experimental Metastasis* 14, no. 2 (1996): 176–86.

25. Webb, Bradley A., Michael Chimenti, Matthew P. Jacobson, and Diane L. Barber. "Dysregulated pH: A perfect storm for cancer progression." *Nature Reviews Cancer* 11, no. 9 (2011): 671.

26. "Hidden in Plain Sight." SugarScience: The Unsweetened Truth. University of California, San Francisco. Accessed on April 24, 2016, http://www.sugarscience .org/hidden-in-plain-sight/.

CHAPTER 5

1. Tryon, Matthew S., Kimber L. Stanhope, Elissa S. Epel, Ashley E. Mason, Rashida Brown, Valentina Medici, Peter J. Havel, and Kevin D. Laugero. "Excessive sugar consumption may be a difficult habit to break: A view from the brain and body." *Journal of Clinical Endocrinology & Metabolism* 100, no. 6 (2015): 2239–47. http://press. endocrine.org/doi/abs/10.1210/jc.2014-4353#sthash.ioq2HYeF.dpuf.

2. Fishman, AP, RM Berne, and HE Morgan. "By the Numbers." *American Journal of Physiology: Gastrointestinal and Liver Physiology* 241, no. 3 (1981): G197–G198.

3. Konturek, Peter C., T. Brzozowski, and S. J. Konturek. "Stress and the gut: Pathophysiology, clinical consequences, diagnostic approach and treatment options." *Journal of Physiology and Pharmacology* 62, no. 6 (2011): 591–99.

4. Konturek, Brzozowski, and Konturek, "Stress and the gut," 591–99.

5. Dinan, Timothy G., and John F. Cryan. "Regulation of the stress response by the gut microbiota: Implications for psychoneuroendocrinology." *Psychoneuroendocrinology* 37, no. 9 (2012): 1369–78.

6. Manenschijn, Laura, Laura Schaap, N. M. Van Schoor, Suzan van der Pas, G. M. E. E. Peeters, Paul Lips, J. W. Koper, and E. F. C. Van Rossum. "High long-term cortisol levels, measured in scalp hair, are associated with a history of cardiovascular disease." *Journal of Clinical Endocrinology & Metabolism* 98, no. 5 (2013): 2078–83.

7. Holick, Michael F., and Tai C. Chen. "Vitamin D deficiency: A worldwide problem with health consequences." *American Journal of Clinical Nutrition* 87, no. 4 (2008): 1080S–1086S.

8. Krajmalnik-Brown, Rosa, Zehra-Esra Ilhan, Dae-Wook Kang, and John K. DiBaise. "Effects of gut microbes on nutrient absorption and energy regulation." *Nutrition in Clinical Practice* 27, no. 2 (2012): 201–14.

9. Fitzgibbon, Joe. *Feeling Tired All the Time—A Comprehensive Guide to the Common Causes of Fatigue and How to Treat Them: Overcome Your Chronic Tiredness.* 2nd edition. Gill Books, 2001.

10. "Vitamin B12 Deficiency Anemia." Johns Hopkins Medical Health Library. Accessed September 1, 2017, http://www.hopkinsmedicine.org/healthlibrary/con ditions/hematology_and_blood_disorders/anemia_of_b12_deficiency_pernicious_ane mia_85,P00080/.

11. Antoni, Michael H., Dean G. Cruess, Stacy Cruess, Susan Lutgendorf, Mahendra Kumar, Gail Ironson, Nancy Klimas, Mary Ann Fletcher, and Neil Schneiderman. "Cognitive-behavioral stress management intervention effects on anxiety, 24-hr

urinary norepinephrine output, and T-cytotoxic/suppressor cells over time among symptomatic HIV-infected gay men." *Journal of Consulting and Clinical Psychology* 68, no. 1 (2000): 31.

12. Davidson, Richard J., Jon Kabat-Zinn, Jessica Schumacher, Melissa Rosenkranz, Daniel Muller, Saki F. Santorelli, Ferris Urbanowski, Anne Harrington, Katherine Bonus, and John F. Sheridan. "Alterations in brain and immune function produced by mindfulness meditation." *Psychosomatic Medicine* 65, no. 4 (2003): 564–70.

13. Tang, Yi-Yuan, Yinghua Ma, Yaxin Fan, Hongbo Feng, Junhong Wang, Shigang Feng, Qilin Lu, et al. "Central and autonomic nervous system interaction is altered by short-term meditation." *Proceedings of the National Academy of Sciences* 106, no. 22 (2009): 8865–70.

14. Hsiao, Elaine Y., Sara W. McBride, Sophia Hsien, Gil Sharon, Embriette R. Hyde, Tyler McCue, and Julian A. Codelli et al. "The microbiota modulates gut physiology and behavioral abnormalities associated with autism." *Cell* 155, no. 7 (2013): 1451.

15. Schmidt, Kristin, Philip J. Cowen, Catherine J. Harmer, George Tzortzis, Steven Errington, and Philip WJ Burnet. "Prebiotic intake reduces the waking cortisol response and alters emotional bias in healthy volunteers." *Psychopharmacology* 232, no. 10 (2015): 1793–1801.

16. Bravo, Javier A., Paul Forsythe, Marianne V. Chew, Emily Escaravage, Hélène M. Savignac, Timothy G. Dinan, John Bienenstock, and John F. Cryan. "Ingestion of *Lactobacillus* strain regulates emotional behavior and central GABA receptor expression in a mouse via the vagus nerve." *Proceedings of the National Academy of Sciences* 108, no. 38 (2011): 16050–55.

17. Messaoudi, Michaël, Robert Lalonde, Nicolas Violle, Hervé Javelot, Didier Desor, Amine Nejdi, Jean-François Bisson, et al. "Assessment of psychotropic-like properties of a probiotic formulation (Lactobacillus helveticus R0052 and Bifidobacterium longum R0175) in rats and human subjects." *British Journal of Nutrition* 105, no. 5 (2011): 755–64.

18. Mullin, Gerard E. *The Gut Balance Revolution.* New York: Rodale Inc., 2014.

19. Schmidt et al., "Prebiotic intake reduces the waking cortisol response," 1793–1801.

20. Singleton, Omar, Britta K. Hölzel, Mark Vangel, Narayan Brach, James Carmody, and Sara W. Lazar. "Change in brainstem gray matter concentration following a mindfulness-based intervention is correlated with improvement in psychological well-being." *Frontiers in Human Neuroscience* 8 (2014).

21. Goyal, Madhav, Sonal Singh, Erica MS Sibinga, Neda F. Gould, Anastasia Rowland-Seymour, Ritu Sharma, Zackary Berger, et al. "Meditation programs for psychological stress and well-being: A systematic review and meta-analysis." *JAMA Internal Medicine* 174, no. 3 (2014): 357–68.

22. Brook, Robert D., Lawrence J. Appel, Melvyn Rubenfire, Gbenga Ogedegbe, John D. Bisognano, William J. Elliott, Flavio D. Fuchs, et al. "Beyond medications and diet: Alternative approaches to lowering blood pressure." *Hypertension* (2013): HYP-0b013e318293645f.

23. Nidich, Sanford I., Maxwell V. Rainforth, David AF Haaga, John Hagelin, John W. Salerno, Fred Travis, Melissa Tanner, Carolyn Gaylord-King, Sarina Grosswald, and Robert H. Schneider. "A randomized controlled trial on effects of the

Transcendental Meditation program on blood pressure, psychological distress, and coping in young adults." *American Journal of Hypertension* 22, no. 12 (2009): 1326–31.

24. Wetherell, Julie Loebach, Lin Liu, Thomas L. Patterson, Niloofar Afari, Catherine R. Ayers, Steven R. Thorp, Jill A. Stoddard, et al. "Acceptance and commitment therapy for generalized anxiety disorder in older adults: A preliminary report." *Behavior Therapy* 42, no. 1 (2011): 127–34.

25. Wetherell, Julie Loebach, Niloofar Afari, Thomas Rutledge, John T. Sorrell, Jill A. Stoddard, Andrew J. Petkus, Brittany C. Solomon, et al. "A randomized, controlled trial of acceptance and commitment therapy and cognitive-behavioral therapy for chronic pain." *Pain* 152, no. 9 (2011): 2098–2107.

26. Tang et al., "Central and autonomic nervous system interaction is altered by short-term meditation," 8865–70.

CHAPTER 6

1. Bull-Otterson, Lara, Wenke Feng, Irina Kirpich, Yuhua Wang, Xiang Qin, Yanlong Liu, Leila Gobejishvili, et al. "Metagenomic analyses of alcohol induced pathogenic alterations in the intestinal microbiome and the effect of Lactobacillus rhamnosus GG treatment." *PLoS One* 8, no. 1 (2013): e53028.

2. Parlesak, Alexandr, Christian Schäfer, Tatjana Schütz, J. Christian Bode, and Christiane Bode. "Increased intestinal permeability to macromolecules and endotoxemia in patients with chronic alcohol abuse in different stages of alcohol-induced liver disease." *Journal of Hepatology* 32, no. 5 (2000): 742–47.

3. Murray, Michael T., and Joseph E. Pizzorno. *Encyclopedia of Natural Medicine*. 3rd edition. Atria Books, 2012.

4. Schley, P. D., and C. J. Field. "The immune-enhancing effects of dietary fibres and prebiotics." *British Journal of Nutrition* 87, no. S2 (2002): S221–S230.

5. Avena, Nicole M., Kristin A. Long, and Bartley G. Hoebel. "Sugar-dependent rats show enhanced responding for sugar after abstinence: Evidence of a sugar deprivation effect." *Physiology & Behavior* 84, no. 3 (2005): 359–62.

6. Lally, Phillippa, and Benjamin Gardner. "Promoting habit formation." *Health Psychology Review* 7, suppl. 1 (2013): S137–S158.

7. Challem, J. and R. Hunninghake. *Stop Prediabetes Now*. Hoboken, NJ: John Wiley & Sons, 2007. See more at https://www.naturalgrocers.com/nutrition-and-health/nutrition-library/nutrition-article/maintain-healthy-blood-sugar-balance-with-food/#_edn23.

8. Jang, HJ, SD Ridgeway, and JA Kim. "Effects of the green tea polyphenol and epigallocatechin-3-gallate on high-fat diet-induced insulin resistance and endothelial dysfunction." *American Journal of Physiology—Endocrinology and Metabolism* 305, no. 12 (2013): E1444–51.

9. Erejuwa, OO, SA Sulaiman, and MS Wahab. "Oligosaccharides might contribute to the antidiabetic effect of honey: A review of the literature." *Molecules* 17, no. 1 (2011): 248–66.

10. Nielsen, Forrest H. "Ultratrace minerals." *Modern Nutrition in Health and Disease* 8 (1999).

11. Saarinen, K., J. Jantunen, and T. Haahtela. "Birch pollen honey for birch pollen allergy—a randomized controlled pilot study." *International Archives of Allergy and Immunology* 155, no. 2 (2011): 160–66.

12. Swithers, Susan E. "Artificial sweeteners produce the counterintuitive effect of inducing metabolic derangements." *Trends in Endocrinology & Metabolism* 24, no. 9 (2013): 431–41.

13. Swithers, Susan E., and Terry L. Davidson. "A role for sweet taste: Calorie predictive relations in energy regulation by rats." *Behavioral Neuroscience* 122, no. 1 (2008): 161.

14. Chen, W. J., J. Wang, X. Y. Qi, and B. J. Xie. "The antioxidant activities of natural sweeteners, mogrosides, from fruits of Siraitia grosvenori." *International Journal of Food Sciences and Nutrition* 58, no. 7 (2007): 548–56.

15. Xu, Q., S. Y. Chen, L. D. Deng, L. P. Feng, L. Z. Huang, and R. R. Yu. "Antioxidant effect of mogrosides against oxidative stress induced by palmitic acid in mouse insulinoma NIT-1 cells." *Brazilian Journal of Medical and Biological Research* 46, no. 11 (2013): 949–55.

16. Ukiya, Motohiko, Toshihiro Akihisa, Harukuni Tokuda, Masakazu Toriumi, Teruo Mukainaka, Norihiro Banno, Yumiko Kimura, Jun-ichi Hasegawa, and Hoyoku Nishino. "Inhibitory effects of cucurbitane glycosides and other triterpenoids from the fruit of *Momordica grosvenori* on Epstein-Barr virus early antigen induced by tumor promoter 12-O-tetradecanoylphorbol-13-acetate." *Journal of Agricultural and Food Chemistry* 50, no. 23 (2002): 6710–15.

CHAPTER 7

1. "Harvard Medical School glycemic index and glycemic load for 100+ foods." Harvard Health Publications. Accessed December 12, 2017, https://www.health.harvard.edu/diseases-and-conditions/glycemic-index-and-glycemic-load-for-100-foods.

2. Cordain, Loren, S. Boyd Eaton, Anthony Sebastian, Neil Mann, Staffan Lindeberg, Bruce A. Watkins, James H. O'Keefe, and Janette Brand-Miller. "Origins and evolution of the Western diet: Health implications for the 21st century." *American Journal of Clinical Nutrition* 81, no. 2 (2005): 341–54.

3. De Punder, Karin, and Leo Pruimboom. "The dietary intake of wheat and other cereal grains and their role in inflammation." *Nutrients* 5, no. 3 (2013): 771–87. doi:10.3390/nu5030771.

4. Drago et al. "Gliadin, zonulin, and gut permeability: Effects on celiac and non-celiac intestinal mucosa and intestinal cell lines." *Scandinavian Journal of Gastroenterology* 41 (2006): 408–19.

5. Neuhausen, Susan L., Linda Steele, Sarah Ryan, Maryam Mousavi, Marie Pinto, Kathryn E. Osann, Pamela Flodman, and John J. Zone. "Co-occurrence of celiac dis-

ease and other autoimmune diseases in celiacs and their first-degree relatives." *Journal of Autoimmunity* 31, no. 2 (2008): 160–65.

6. Benbrook, Charles M. "Trends in glyphosate herbicide use in the United States and globally." *Environmental Sciences Europe* 28, no. 1 (2016): 3.

7. "Internal EPA documents show scramble for data on Monsanto's Roundup herbicide." *Huffington Post*. Accessed September 14, 2017, https://www.huffing tonpost.com/entry/internal-epa-documents-show-scramble-for-data-on-monsantos_ us_5988dd73e4b030f0e267c6cd.

8. Samsel, Anthony, and Stephanie Seneff. "Glyphosate's suppression of cyto-chrome P450 enzymes and amino acid biosynthesis by the gut microbiome: Pathways to modern diseases." *Entropy* 15, no. 4 (2013): 1416–63.

9. Samsel, Anthony, and Stephanie Seneff. "Glyphosate, pathways to modern diseases II: Celiac sprue and gluten intolerance." *Interdisciplinary Toxicology* 6, no. 4 (2013): 159–84.

10. Rubio-Tapia, Alberto, Robert A. Kyle, Edward L. Kaplan, Dwight R. Johnson, William Page, Frederick Erdtmann, Tricia L. Brantner, et al. "Increased prevalence and mortality in undiagnosed celiac disease." *Gastroenterology* 137, no. 1 (2009): 88–93.

11. Samsel and Seneff, "Glyphosate, pathways to modern diseases II."

12. Samsel and Seneff, "Glyphosate, pathways to modern diseases II."

13. Senapati, T., A. K. Mukerjee, and A. R. Ghosh. "Observations on the effect of glyphosate based herbicide on ultra structure (SEM) and enzymatic activity in different regions of alimentary canal and gill of Channa punctatus (Bloch)." *Journal of Crop and Weed* 5, no. 1 (2009): 236–45.

14. Williams, Gary M., Robert Kroes, and Ian C. Munro. "Safety evaluation and risk assessment of the herbicide Roundup and its active ingredient, glyphosate, for humans." *Regulatory Toxicology and Pharmacology* 31, no. 2 (2000): 117–65.

15. Fritschi, L., J. McLaughlin, C. M. Sergi, G. M. Calaf, F. Le Curieux, F. Forast-iere, H. Kromhout, et al. "Carcinogenicity of tetrachlorvinphos, parathion, malathion, diazinon, and glyphosate." *Red* 114, no. 2 (2015).

16. Hoppe, H. W. "Determination of glyphosate residues in human urine samples from 18 European countries." Medical Laboratory Bremen, D-28357 Bremen, Ger-many (2013).

17. Lindfors, K., T. Blomqvist, K. Juuti-Uusitalo, S. Stenman, J. Venäläinen, M. Mäki, and K. Kaukinen. "Live probiotic Bifidobacterium lactis bacteria inhibit the toxic effects induced by wheat gliadin in epithelial cell culture." *Clinical & Experimental Immunology* 152, no. 3 (2008): 552–58.

18. Whorwell, Peter J., Linda Altringer, Jorge Morel, Yvonne Bond, Duane Char-bonneau, Liam O'Mahony, Barry Kiely, Fergus Shanahan, and Eamonn MM Quig-ley. "Efficacy of an encapsulated probiotic Bifidobacterium infantis 35624 in women with irritable bowel syndrome." *American Journal of Gastroenterology* 101, no. 7 (2006): 1581–90.

19. Rizzello, CG, M De Angelis, R Di Cagno, et al. "Highly efficient gluten degradation by lactobacilli and fungal proteases during food processing: New per-spectives for celiac disease." *Applied and Environmental Microbiology* 73, no. 14 (2007): 4499–4507. doi:10.1128/AEM.00260-07.

CHAPTER 8

1. Nestle, Marion. *Food Politics: How the Food Industry Influences Nutrition and Health.* Vol. 3. Berkeley: University of California Press, 2013.

2. Danby, F. William. "Nutrition and acne." *Clinics in Dermatology* 28, no. 6 (2010): 598–604.

3. Nilsson, Mikael, Marianne Stenberg, Anders H. Frid, Jens J. Holst, and Inger ME Björck. "Glycemia and insulinemia in healthy subjects after lactose-equivalent meals of milk and other food proteins: The role of plasma amino acids and incretins." *The American Journal of Clinical Nutrition* 80, no. 5 (2004): 1246–53.

4. Dandona, Paresh, Ahmad Aljada, and Arindam Bandyopadhyay. "Inflammation: The link between insulin resistance, obesity and diabetes." *Trends in Immunology* 25, no. 1 (2004): 4–7.

5. Vane, John, and Regina Botting. "Inflammation and the mechanism of action of anti-inflammatory drugs." *FASEB Journal* 1, no. 2 (1987): 89–96.

6. Danby, F. William (Bill). "Acne: Diet and acnegenesis." *Indian Dermatology Online Journal* 2, no. 1 (2011): 2.

7. Ismail, Noor Hasnani, Zahara Abdul Manaf, and Noor Zalmy Azizan. "High glycemic load diet, milk and ice cream consumption are related to acne vulgaris in Malaysian young adults: A case control study." *BMC Dermatology* 12, no. 1 (2012): 13.

8. Turner, Andrew G., Paul H. Anderson, and Howard A. Morris. "Vitamin D and bone health." *Scandinavian Journal of Clinical and Laboratory Investigation* 72, suppl. 243 (2012): 65–72.

9. Michaëlsson, Karl, Alicja Wolk, Sophie Langenskiöld, Samar Basu, Eva Warensjö Lemming, Håkan Melhus, and Liisa Byberg. "Milk intake and risk of mortality and fractures in women and men: Cohort studies." *BMJ* 349 (2014): g6015.

10. Lanou, Amy Joy, Susan E. Berkow, and Neal D. Barnard. "Calcium, dairy products, and bone health in children and young adults: A reevaluation of the evidence." *Pediatrics* 115, no. 3 (2005): 736–43.

11. Chen et al. "Dairy consumption and risk of type 2 diabetes: 3 cohorts of US adults and an updated meta-analysis." *BMC Medicine* 12 (2014): 215. http://www.biomedcentral.com/1741-7015/12/215.

12. "Milk Production 2012." U.S. Department of Agriculture, National Agriculture Statistics Service. July 19, 2012.

13. Cancer.org. "Recombinant Bovine Growth Hormone." Accessed July 22, 2015, http://www.cancer.org/cancer/cancercauses/othercarcinogens/athome/recombinant-bovine-growth-hormone.

14. Raloff, J. "Hormones: Here's the beef: Environmental concerns reemerge over steroids given to livestock." *Science News* 161, no 1 (2002).

15. Magis, D. C., B. J. Jandrain, and A. J. Scheen. "Alcohol, insulin sensitivity and diabetes." *Revue Medicale de Liege* 58, no. 7–8 (2002): 501–7.

16. Townshend, Julia, and Theodora Duka. "Attentional bias associated with alcohol cues: Differences between heavy and occasional social drinkers." *Psychopharmacology* 157, no. 1 (2001): 67–74.

17. Parlesak, Alexandr, Christian Schäfer, Tatjana Schütz, J. Christian Bode, and Christiane Bode. "Increased intestinal permeability to macromolecules and endotox-

emia in patients with chronic alcohol abuse in different stages of alcohol-induced liver disease." *Journal of Hepatology* 32, no. 5 (2000): 742–47.

18. Mutlu, Ece A., Patrick M. Gillevet, Huzefa Rangwala, Masoumeh Sikaroodi, Ammar Naqvi, Phillip A. Engen, Mary Kwasny, Cynthia K. Lau, and Ali Keshavarzian. "Colonic microbiome is altered in alcoholism." *American Journal of Physiology–Gastrointestinal and Liver Physiology* 302, no. 9 (2012): G966–G978.

19. Bull-Otterson, Lara, Wenke Feng, Irina Kirpich, Yuhua Wang, Xiang Qin, Yanlong Liu, Leila Gobejishvili, et al. "Metagenomic analyses of alcohol induced pathogenic alterations in the intestinal microbiome and the effect of Lactobacillus rhamnosus GG treatment." *PLoS One* 8, no. 1 (2013): e53028.

20. Bode, Christiane, and J. Christian Bode. "Effect of alcohol consumption on the gut." *Best Practice & Research Clinical Gastroenterology* 17, no. 4 (2003): 575–92.

21. Bode and Bode, "Effect of alcohol consumption on the gut."

22. Bode and Bode, "Effect of alcohol consumption on the gut."

CHAPTER 9

1. Grazul, Hannah, L. Leann Kanda, and David Gondek. "Impact of probiotic supplements on microbiome diversity following antibiotic treatment of mice." *Gut Microbes* 7, no. 2 (2016): 101–14.

2. Niness, Kathy R. "Inulin and oligofructose: What are they?" *Journal of Nutrition* 129, no. 7 (1999): 1402S–1406S.

3. Rabiu, Bodun A., and Glenn R. Gibson. "Carbohydrates: A limit on bacterial diversity within the colon." *Biological Reviews* 77, no. 3 (2002): 443–53.

4. Wong, Julia MW, Russell De Souza, Cyril WC Kendall, Azadeh Emam, and David JA Jenkins. "Colonic health: Fermentation and short chain fatty acids." *Journal of Clinical Gastroenterology* 40, no. 3 (2006): 235–43.

5. Bourassa, Megan W., Ishraq Alim, Scott J. Bultman, and Rajiv R. Ratan. "Butyrate, neuroepigenetics and the gut microbiome: Can a high fiber diet improve brain health?" *Neuroscience Letters* 625 (2016): 56–63.

6. Bourassa et al., "Butyrate, neuroepigenetics and the gut microbiome," 56–63.

7. Ahn, Y. J., S. Sakanaka, M. J. Kim, T. Kawamura, T. Fujisawa, and T. Mitsuoka. "Effect of green tea extract on growth of intestinal bacteria." *Microbial Ecology in Health and Disease* 3, no. 6 (1990): 335–38.

8. Lee, Hui Cheng, Andrew M. Jenner, Chin Seng Low, and Yuan Kun Lee. "Effect of tea phenolics and their aromatic fecal bacterial metabolites on intestinal microbiota." *Research in Microbiology* 157, no. 9 (2006): 876–84.

9. Chen, Lei, William CS Tai, and WL Wendy Hsiao. "Dietary saponins from four popular herbal teas exert prebiotic-like effects on gut microbiota in C57BL/6 mice." *Journal of Functional Foods* 17 (2015): 892–902.

10. Jin, Jong-Sik, Mutsumi Touyama, Takayoshi Hisada, and Yoshimi Benno. "Effects of green tea consumption on human fecal microbiota with special reference to Bifidobacterium species." *Microbiology and Immunology* 56, no. 11 (2012): 729–39.

11. Şanlier, Nevin, Büşra Başar Gökcen, and Aybüke Ceyhun Sezgin. "Health benefits of fermented foods." *Critical Reviews in Food Science and Nutrition* (2017): 1–22.

12. Şanlier, Gökcen, and Sezgin, "Health benefits of fermented foods," 1–22.

13. Choi, In Hwa, Jeong Sook Noh, Ji-Sook Han, Hyun Ju Kim, Eung-Soo Han, and Yeong Ok Song. "Kimchi, a fermented vegetable, improves serum lipid profiles in healthy young adults: Randomized clinical trial." *Journal of Medicinal Food* 16, no. 3 (2013): 223–29.

14. Hertzler, Steven R., and Shannon M. Clancy. "Kefir improves lactose digestion and tolerance in adults with lactose maldigestion." *Journal of the American Dietetic Association* 103, no. 5 (2003): 582–87.

15. Axe, Josh. *Eat Dirt: Why Leaky Gut May Be the Root Cause of Your Health Problems and 5 Surprising Steps to Cure It*. HarperCollins Publishers, 2016.

16. Henning, Susanne M., Yanjun Zhang, Navindra P. Seeram, Ru-Po Lee, Piwen Wang, Susan Bowerman, and David Heber. "Antioxidant capacity and phytochemical content of herbs and spices in dry, fresh and blended herb paste form." *International Journal of Food Sciences and Nutrition* 62, no. 3 (2011): 219–25.

17. Tuohy, Kieran M., Lorenza Conterno, Mattia Gasperotti, and Roberto Viola. "Up-regulating the human intestinal microbiome using whole plant foods, polyphenols, and/or fiber." *Journal of Agricultural and Food Chemistry* 60, no. 36 (2012): 8776–82.

18. Liju, Vijayasteltar B., Kottarapat Jeena, and Ramadasan Kuttan. "Gastroprotective activity of essential oils from turmeric and ginger." *Journal of Basic and Clinical Physiology and Pharmacology* 26, no. 1 (2015): 95–103.

19. "The Overuse of Antibiotics in Farm Animals Threatens Public Health." Consumers Union: Policy & Action from Consumer Reports, Accessed September 29, 2017, http://consumersunion.org/pdf/Overuse_of_Antibiotics_On_Farms.pdf.

20. Guidos, Robert, J. "IDSA public policy: Combating antimicrobial resistance: Policy recommendations to save lives." *Clinical Infectious Diseases* 52, suppl. 5 (2011): S397.

21. Ebbesson, SO, PM Risica, LO Ebbesson, JM Kennish, and ME Tejero. "Omega-3 fatty acids improve glucose tolerance and components of the metabolic syndrome in Alaskan Eskimos: The Alaskan Siberia project." *International Journal of Circumpolar Health* 64, no. 4 (2005): 396–408.

22. Hutchins, H, and CP Vega. "Symposium Highlights—Omega-3 fatty acids: Recommendations for therapeutics and prevention." *Medscape General Medicine* 7, no. 4 (2005): 18. See more at: https://www.naturalgrocers.com/nutrition-and-health/nutrition-library/nutrition-article/maintain-healthy-blood-sugar-balance-with-food/#_edn10.

23. Challem J, and R Hunninghake. *Stop Prediabetes Now*. Hoboken, NJ: John Wiley & Sons, 2007.

24. Remer, Thomas, and Friedrich Manz. "Potential renal acid load of foods and its influence on urine pH." *Journal of the American Dietetic Association* 95, no. 7 (1995): 791–97.

25. Smith, Bob L. "Organic foods vs. supermarket foods: Element levels." *Journal of Applied Nutrition* 45, no. 1 (1993): 35–39.

26. Lopez-Ridaura, Ruy, Walter C. Willett, Eric B. Rimm, Simin Liu, Meir J. Stampfer, JoAnn E. Manson, and Frank B. Hu. "Magnesium intake and risk of type 2 diabetes in men and women." *Diabetes Care* 27, no. 1 (2004): 134–40.

27. Remer and Manz. "Potential renal acid load of foods and its influence on urine pH," 791–97.

28. Kang, Dezhi, Baochen Shi, Marie C. Erfe, Noah Craft, and Huiying Li. "Vitamin B12 modulates the transcriptome of the skin microbiota in acne pathogenesis." *Science Translational Medicine* 7, no. 293 (2015): 293ra103.

29. Jansen, T., R. Romiti, A. Kreuter, and P. Altmeyer. "Rosacea fulminans triggered by high-dose vitamins B6 and B12." *Journal of the European Academy of Dermatology and Venereology* 15, no. 5 (2001): 484–85.

30. Nestle, Marion. "Diet, Life-style, and Mortality in China: A Study of the Characteristics of 65 Chinese Counties." *BioScience* 41, no. 10 (1991): 725–27.

31. Minich, Deanna M., and Jeffrey S. Bland. "Acid-alkaline balance: Role in chronic disease and detoxification." *Alternative Therapies in Health and Medicine* 13, no. 4 (2007): 62.

32. Caballero, Benjamin. *Encyclopedia of Human Nutrition*. Academic Press, 2012.

CHAPTER 10

1. Aslam, Muhammad N., Tejaswi Paruchuri, Narasimharao Bhagavathula, and James Varani. "A mineral-rich red algae extract inhibits polyp formation and inflammation in the gastrointestinal tract of mice on a high-fat diet." *Integrative Cancer Therapies* 9, no. 1 (2010): 93–99.

2. Maron, David J. "Flavonoids for reduction of atherosclerotic risk." *Current Atherosclerosis Reports* 6, no. 1 (2004): 73–78.

3. Johnson, S. "The multifaceted and widespread pathology of magnesium deficiency." *Medical Hypotheses* 56, no. 2 (2001): 163–70.

Bibliography

Ackerman, Jennifer. "The ultimate social network." *Scientific American* 306, no. 6 (2012): 36–43.

"Advertising spending of the food and beverage industry in the United States in 2013, by medium (in thousand U.S. dollars)." Statista: The Statistics Portal. Accessed December 14, 2017, https://www.statista.com/statistics/319053/food-beverage-ad-spend- medium/.

Aeberli, Isabelle, Philipp A. Gerber, Michel Hochuli, Sibylle Kohler, Sarah R. Haile, Ioanna Gouni-Berthold, Heiner K. Berthold, Giatgen A. Spinas, and Kaspar Berneis. "Low to moderate sugar-sweetened beverage consumption impairs glucose and lipid metabolism and promotes inflammation in healthy young men: A randomized controlled trial." *The American Journal of Clinical Nutrition* 94, no. 2 (2011): 479–85.

Ahmed, Serge H. "Is sugar as addictive as cocaine?" *Food and Addiction: A Comprehensive Handbook* (2012): 231–37.

Ahn, Y. J., S. Sakanaka, M. J. Kim, T. Kawamura, T. Fujisawa, and T. Mitsuoka. "Effect of green tea extract on growth of intestinal bacteria." *Microbial Ecology in Health and Disease* 3, no. 6 (1990): 335–38.

Alcock, Joe, Carlo C. Maley, and C. Aktipis. "Is eating behavior manipulated by the gastrointestinal microbiota? Evolutionary pressures and potential mechanisms." *Bioessays* 36, no. 10 (2014): 940–49.

Antoni, Michael H., Dean G. Cruess, Stacy Cruess, Susan Lutgendorf, Mahendra Kumar, Gail Ironson, Nancy Klimas, Mary Ann Fletcher, and Neil Schneiderman. "Cognitive-behavioral stress management intervention effects on anxiety, 24-hr urinary norepinephrine output, and T-cytotoxic/suppressor cells over time among symptomatic HIV-infected gay men." *Journal of Consulting and Clinical Psychology* 68, no. 1 (2000): 31.

"Are Your Health Problems Yeast Connected?" The Yeast Connection. Accessed September 15, 2016, http://www.yeastconnection.com.

Aslam, Muhammad N., Tejaswi Paruchuri, Narasimharao Bhagavathula, and James Varani. "A mineral-rich red algae extract inhibits polyp formation and inflammation in the gastrointestinal tract of mice on a high-fat diet." *Integrative Cancer Therapies* 9, no. 1 (2010): 93–99.

Avena, Nicole M., Kristin A. Long, and Bartley G. Hoebel. "Sugar-dependent rats show enhanced responding for sugar after abstinence: Evidence of a sugar deprivation effect." *Physiology & Behavior* 84, no. 3 (2005): 359–62.

Avena, Nicole M., Pedro Rada, and Bartley G. Hoebel. "Evidence for sugar addiction: Behavioral and neurochemical effects of intermittent, excessive sugar intake." *Neuroscience & Biobehavioral Reviews* 32, no. 1 (2008): 20–39.

Axe, Josh. *Eat Dirt: Why Leaky Gut May Be the Root Cause of Your Health Problems and 5 Surprising Ways to Cure It.* HarperCollins Publishers, 2016.

Bailey, L. Charles, Christopher B. Forrest, Peixin Zhang, Thomas M. Richards, Alice Livshits, and Patricia A. DeRusso. "Association of antibiotics in infancy with early childhood obesity." *JAMA Pediatrics* 168, no. 11 (2014): 1063–69.

Benbrook, Charles M. "Trends in glyphosate herbicide use in the United States and globally." *Environmental Sciences Europe* 28, no. 1 (2016): 3.

Bengmark, S. "Nutrition of the critically ill—a 21st century perspective." *Nutrients* 5 (2013): 162–207.

"Biologists ID Defense Mechanism of Leading Fungal Pathogen." *EurekAlert!* Accessed October 21, 2017, http://www.eurekalert.org/pub_releases/2004-06/ru-bid 062504.php.

Bode, Christiane, and J. Christian Bode. "Effect of alcohol consumption on the gut." *Best Practice & Research Clinical Gastroenterology* 17, no. 4 (2003): 575–92.

Bourassa, Megan W., Ishraq Alim, Scott J. Bultman, and Rajiv R. Ratan. "Butyrate, neuroepigenetics and the gut microbiome: Can a high fiber diet improve brain health?" *Neuroscience Letters* 625 (2016): 56–63.

Bravo, Javier A., Paul Forsythe, Marianne V. Chew, Emily Escaravage, Hélène M. Savignac, Timothy G. Dinan, John Bienenstock, and John F. Cryan. "Ingestion of *Lactobacillus* strain regulates emotional behavior and central GABA receptor expression in a mouse via the vagus nerve." *Proceedings of the National Academy of Sciences* 108, no. 38 (2011): 16050–16055.

Brook, Robert D., Lawrence J. Appel, Melvyn Rubenfire, Gbenga Ogedegbe, John D. Bisognano, William J. Elliott, Flavio D. Fuchs, et al. "Beyond medications and diet: Alternative approaches to lowering blood pressure." *Hypertension* (2013): HYP-0b013e318293645f.

Bull-Otterson, Lara, Wenke Feng, Irina Kirpich, Yuhua Wang, Xiang Qin, Yanlong Liu, Leila Gobejishvili, et al. "Metagenomic analyses of alcohol induced pathogenic alterations in the intestinal microbiome and the effect of Lactobacillus rhamnosus GG treatment." *PLoS One* 8, no. 1 (2013): e53028.

Caballero, Benjamin. *Encyclopedia of Human Nutrition.* Academic Press, 2012.

Carrasco, Andrés. "Teratogenesis by glyphosate based herbicides and other pesticides. Relationship with the retinoic acid pathway." *GMLS* 2012 (2013): 24.

Challem J, and R Hunninghake. *Stop Prediabetes Now.* Hoboken, NJ: John Wiley & Sons, 2007.

Chatterjee, Soumya, Sandy Park, Kimberly Low, Yuthana Kong, and Mark Pimentel. "The degree of breath methane production in IBS correlates with the severity of constipation." *American Journal of Gastroenterology* 102, no. 4 (2007): 837.

Chedid, Victor, Sameer Dhalla, John O. Clarke, Bani Chander Roland, Kerry B. Dunbar, Joyce Koh, Edmundo Justino, Eric Tomakin RN, and Gerard E. Mullin. "Herbal therapy is equivalent to rifaximin for the treatment of small intestinal bacterial overgrowth." *Global Advances in Health and Medicine* 3, no. 3 (2014): 16–24.

Chen et al. "Dairy consumption and risk of type 2 diabetes: 3 cohorts of US adults and an updated meta-analysis." *BMC Medicine* 12 (2014): 215. http://www.biomedcen tral.com/1741-7015/12/215.

Chen, Lei, William CS Tai, and WL Wendy Hsiao. "Dietary saponins from four popular herbal teas exert prebiotic-like effects on gut microbiota in C57BL/6 mice." *Journal of Functional Foods* 17 (2015): 892–902.

Chen, W. J., J. Wang, X. Y. Qi, and B. J. Xie. "The antioxidant activities of natural sweeteners, mogrosides, from fruits of Siraitia grosvenori." *International Journal of Food Sciences and Nutrition* 58, no. 7 (2007): 548–56.

Choi, In Hwa, Jeong Sook Noh, Ji-Sook Han, Hyun Ju Kim, Eung-Soo Han, and Yeong Ok Song. "Kimchi, a fermented vegetable, improves serum lipid profiles in healthy young adults: Randomized clinical trial." *Journal of Medicinal Food* 16, no. 3 (2013): 223–29.

Colantuoni, Carlo, Pedro Rada, Joseph McCarthy, Caroline Patten, Nicole M. Avena, Andrew Chadeayne, and Bartley G. Hoebel. "Evidence that intermittent, excessive sugar intake causes endogenous opioid dependence." *Obesity* 10, no. 6 (2002): 478–88.

Cordain, Loren, S. Boyd Eaton, Anthony Sebastian, Neil Mann, Staffan Lindeberg, Bruce A. Watkins, James H. O'Keefe, and Janette Brand-Miller. "Origins and evolution of the Western diet: Health implications for the 21st century." *American Journal of Clinical Nutrition* 81, no. 2 (2005): 341–54.

Cotten, C. Michael, Sarah Taylor, Barbara Stoll, Ronald N. Goldberg, Nellie I. Hansen, Pablo J. Sánchez, Namasivayam Ambalavanan, and Daniel K. Benjamin. "Prolonged duration of initial empirical antibiotic treatment is associated with increased rates of necrotizing enterocolitis and death for extremely low birth weight infants." *Pediatrics* 123, no. 1 (2009): 58–66.

Danby, F. William (Bill). "Acne: Diet and acnegenesis." *Indian Dermatology Online Journal* 2, no. 1 (2011): 2.

Danby, F. William. "Nutrition and acne." *Clinics in Dermatology* 28, no. 6 (2010): 598–604.

Dandona, Paresh, Ahmad Aljada, and Arindam Bandyopadhyay. "Inflammation: The link between insulin resistance, obesity and diabetes." *Trends in Immunology* 25, no. 1 (2004): 4–7.

David, LA et al. "Diet rapidly and reproducibly alters the human gut microbiome." *Nature* 505, no. 7484 (2014): 559–63. doi: 10.1038/nature12820.

Davidson, Richard J., Jon Kabat-Zinn, Jessica Schumacher, Melissa Rosenkranz, Daniel Muller, Saki F. Santorelli, Ferris Urbanowski, Anne Harrington, Katherine Bonus, and John F. Sheridan. "Alterations in brain and immune function produced by mindfulness meditation." *Psychosomatic Medicine* 65, no. 4 (2003): 564–70.

De Punder, Karin, and Leo Pruimboom. "The dietary intake of wheat and other cereal grains and their role in inflammation." *Nutrients* 5, no. 3 (2013): 771–87. doi:10.3390/nu5030771.

Dethlefsen, Les, and David A. Relman. "Incomplete recovery and individualized responses of the human distal gut microbiota to repeated antibiotic perturbation." *Proceedings of the National Academy of Sciences* 108, suppl. 1 (2011): 4554–61.

Dinan, Timothy G., and John F. Cryan. "Regulation of the stress response by the gut microbiota: Implications for psychoneuroendocrinology." *Psychoneuroendocrinology* 37, no. 9 (2012): 1369–78.

Drago et al. "Gliadin, zonulin, and gut permeability: Effects on celiac and non-celiac intestinal mucosa and intestinal cell lines." *Scandinavian Journal of Gastroenterology* 41 (2006): 408–19.

Dupont, PF. "Candida albicans, the opportunist. A cellular and molecular perspective." *Journal of the American Podiatric Medical Association* 85, no. 2 (1995): 104–15. http://www.ncbi.nlm.nih.gov/pubmed/7877106.

Ebbesson, SO, PM Risica, LO Ebbesson, JM Kennish, and ME Tejero. "Omega-3 fatty acids improve glucose tolerance and components of the metabolic syndrome in Alaskan Eskimos: The Alaskan Siberia project." *International Journal of Circumpolar Health* 64, no. 4 (2005): 396–408.

Erejuwa, OO, SA Sulaiman, and MS Wahab. "Oligosaccharides might contribute to the antidiabetic effect of honey: A review of the literature." *Molecules* 17, no. 1 (2011): 248–66.

Fan, Di, Laura A. Coughlin, Megan M. Neubauer, Jiwoong Kim, Min Soo Kim, Xiaowei Zhan, Tiffany R. Simms-Waldrip, Yang Xie, Lora V. Hooper, and Andrew Y. Koh. "Activation of HIF-1α and LL-37 by commensal bacteria inhibits *Candida albicans* colonization." *Nature Medicine* 21, no. 7 (2015): 808.

Farias, MM, AM Cuevas, and F Rodriguez. "Set-point theory and obesity." *Metabolic Syndrome and Related Disorders* 9 (2011): 85–89.

"Finding a single mechanism for hypertension, insulin resistance, and immune suppression." UC San Diego Jacobs School of Engineering. Accessed on July 14, 2017, http://jacobsschool.ucsd.edu/news/news_releases/release.sfe?id=744.

Fishman, AP, RM Berne, and HE Morgan. "By the Numbers." *American Journal of Physiology: Gastrointestinal and Liver Physiology* 241, no. 3 (1981): G197–G198.

Fitzgibbon, Joe. *Feeling Tired All the Time—A Comprehensive Guide to the Common Causes of Fatigue and How to Treat Them: Overcome Your Chronic Tiredness*. 2nd edition. Gill Books, 2001.

Frank, Daniel N., and Norman R. Pace. "Gastrointestinal microbiology enters the metagenomics era." *Current Opinion in Gastroenterology* 24, no. 1 (2008): 4–10.

Fritschi, L., J. McLaughlin, C. M. Sergi, G. M. Calaf, F. Le Curieux, F. Forastiere, H. Kromhout, et al. "Carcinogenicity of tetrachlorvinphos, parathion, malathion, diazinon, and glyphosate." *Red* 114, no. 2 (2015).

Ghosh, Sanjoy, Erin Molcan, Daniella DeCoffe, Chaunbin Dai, and Deanna L. Gibson. "Diets rich in n-6 PUFA induce intestinal microbial dysbiosis in aged mice." *British Journal of Nutrition* 110, no. 3 (2013): 515–23.

Gillies, RJ, and Mary JC Hendrix. "Acidic pH enhances the invasive behavior of human melanoma cells." *Clinical & Experimental Metastasis* 14, no. 2 (1996): 176–86.

Gleason, Julie E., Ahmad Galaleldeen, Ryan L. Peterson, Alexander B. Taylor, Stephen P. Holloway, Jessica Waninger-Saroni, Brendan P. Cormack, Diane E. Cabelli, P. John Hart, and Valeria Cizewski Culotta. "Candida albicans SOD5 represents the prototype of an unprecedented class of Cu-only superoxide dismutases required for pathogen defense." *Proceedings of the National Academy of Sciences* 111, no. 16 (2014): 5866–71.

"Glycemic Index and Diabetes."American Diabetes Association. Accessed September 3, 2017, http://www.diabetes.org/food-and-fitness/food/what-can-i-eat/under standing-carbohydrates/glycemic-index-and-diabetes.html?referrer=https://www .google.com/.

"Glyphosate issue paper: Evaluation of carcinogenic potential." EPA's Office of Pesticide Programs. September 12, 2016.

Goyal, Madhav, Sonal Singh, Erica MS Sibinga, Neda F. Gould, Anastasia Rowland-Seymour, Ritu Sharma, Zackary Berger, et al. "Meditation programs for psychological stress and well-being: A systematic review and meta-analysis." *JAMA Internal Medicine* 174, no. 3 (2014): 357–68.

Grazul, Hannah, L. Leann Kanda, and David Gondek. "Impact of probiotic supplements on microbiome diversity following antibiotic treatment of mice." *Gut Microbes* 7, no. 2 (2016): 101–14.

Grice, E. A., and J. A. Segre. "The human microbiome: Our second genome." *Annual Review of Genomics and Human Genetics* 13 (2012): 151–70. http://doi.org/10.1146/annurev-genom-090711-163814.

Grün, Felix, and Bruce Blumberg. "Environmental obesogens: Organotins and endocrine disruption via nuclear receptor signaling." *Endocrinology* 147, no. 6 (2006): s50–s55.

Guidos, Robert, J. "IDSA public policy: Combating antimicrobial resistance: Policy recommendations to save lives." *Clinical Infectious Diseases* 52, suppl. 5 (2011): S397.

"Harvard Medical School glycemic index and glycemic load for 100+ foods." Harvard Health Publications. Accessed December 12, 2017, https://www.health.harvard .edu/diseases-and-conditions/glycemic-index-and-glycemic-load-for-100-foods.

Hemarajata, Peera, and James Versalovic. "Effects of probiotics on gut microbiota: Mechanisms of intestinal immunomodulation and neuromodulation." *Therapeutic Advances in Gastroenterology* 6, no. 1 (2013): 39–51.

Henning, Susanne M., Yanjun Zhang, Navindra P. Seeram, Ru-Po Lee, Piwen Wang, Susan Bowerman, and David Heber. "Antioxidant capacity and phytochemical content of herbs and spices in dry, fresh and blended herb paste form." *International Journal of Food Sciences and Nutrition* 62, no. 3 (2011): 219–25.

Hertzler, Steven R., and Shannon M. Clancy. "Kefir improves lactose digestion and tolerance in adults with lactose maldigestion." *Journal of the American Dietetic Association* 103, no. 5 (2003): 582–87.

"Hidden in Plain Sight." SugarScience: The Unsweetened Truth. University of California, San Francisco. Accessed on April 24, 2016, http://sugarscience.ucsf.edu/hidden- in-plain-sight/.

Holick, Michael F., and Tai C. Chen. "Vitamin D deficiency: A worldwide problem with health consequences." *American Journal of Clinical Nutrition* 87, no. 4 (2008): 1080S–1086S.

Hoppe, H. W. "Determination of glyphosate residues in human urine samples from 18 European countries." Medical Laboratory Bremen, D-28357 Bremen, Germany (2013).

Hostetter, Margaret K. "Handicaps to host defense: Effects of hyperglycemia on C3 and Candida albicans." *Diabetes* 39, no. 3 (1990): 271–75.

"How Much Sugar Are Americans Eating." *Forbes* website. Accessed October 24, 2017, http://www.forbes.com/sites/alicegwalton/2012/08/30/how-much-sugar-are-americans-eating-infographic/.

Hsiao, Elaine Y., Sara W. McBride, Sophia Hsien, Gil Sharon, Embriette R. Hyde, Tyler McCue, Julian A. Codelli, et al. "The microbiota modulates gut physiology and behavioral abnormalities associated with autism." *Cell* 155, no. 7 (2013): 1451.

Hullar, Meredith AJ, and Benjamin C. Fu. "Diet, the gut microbiome, and epigenetics." *Cancer Journal* 20, no. 3 (2014): 170.

Hutchins, H, and CP Vega. "Symposium Highlights—Omega-3 fatty acids: Recommendations for therapeutics and prevention." *Medscape General Medicine* 7, no. 4 (2005): 18.

Ifland, J. R., H. G. Preuss, M. T. Marcus, K. M. Rourke, W. C. Taylor, K. Burau, William Solomon Jacobs, W. Kadish, and G. Manso. "Refined food addiction: A classic substance use disorder." *Medical Hypotheses* 72, no. 5 (2009): 518–26.

Imam, Talha H., MD. "Fungal urinary tract infections." *Merck Manual.* http://www.merckmanuals.com/professional/genitourinary-disorders/urinary-tract-infections-(uti)/fungal-urinary-tract-infections.

"Internal EPA documents show scramble for data on Monsanto's Roundup herbicide." *Huffington Post.* Accessed September 14, 2017, https://www.huffingtonpost.com/entry/internal-epa-documents-show-scramble-for-data-on-monsantos_us_5988dd73e4b030f0e267c6cd.

Ismail, Noor Hasnani, Zahara Abdul Manaf, and Noor Zalmy Azizan. "High glycemic load diet, milk and ice cream consumption are related to acne vulgaris in Malaysian young adults: A case control study." *BMC Dermatology* 12, no. 1 (2012): 13.

Jacobs, Gill, and Joanna Kjaer. *Beat Candida Through Diet: A Complete Dietary Programme for Sufferers of Candidiasis.* Ebury Digital, February 29, 2012.

Jameel, Faizan, Lisa G. Wood, Manohar L. Garg, and Melinda Phang. "Acute effects of feeding fructose, glucose and sucrose on blood lipid levels and systemic inflammation." *Lipids in Health and Disease* 13, no. 1 (2014): 195.

Jang, HJ, SD Ridgeway, and JA Kim. "Effects of the green tea polyphenol and epigallocatechin-3-gallate on high-fat diet-induced insulin resistance and endothelial dysfunction." *American Journal of Physiology–Endocrinology and Metabolism* 305, no. 12 (2013): E1444–51.

Jansen, T., R. Romiti, A. Kreuter, and P. Altmeyer. "Rosacea fulminans triggered by high-dose vitamins B6 and B12." *Journal of the European Academy of Dermatology and Venereology* 15, no. 5 (2001): 484–85.

Jernberg, Cecilia, Sonja Löfmark, Charlotta Edlund, and Janet K. Jansson. "Long-term ecological impacts of antibiotic administration on the human intestinal microbiota." *ISME Journal* 1, no. 1 (2007): 56.

Jin, Jong-Sik, Mutsumi Touyama, Takayoshi Hisada, and Yoshimi Benno. "Effects of green tea consumption on human fecal microbiota with special reference to Bifidobacterium species." *Microbiology and Immunology* 56, no. 11 (2012): 729–39.

Johnson, S. "The multifaceted and widespread pathology of magnesium deficiency." *Medical Hypotheses* 56, no. 2 (2001): 163–70.

Kang, Dezhi, Baochen Shi, Marie C. Erfe, Noah Craft, and Huiying Li. "Vitamin B12 modulates the transcriptome of the skin microbiota in acne pathogenesis." *Science Translational Medicine* 7, no. 293 (2015): 293ra103.

Kauffman, Carol A., John F. Fisher, Jack D. Sobel, and Cheryl A. Newman. "Candida urinary tract infections—diagnosis." *Clinical Infectious Diseases* 52, suppl. 6 (2011): S452–S456.

Konturek, Peter C., T. Brzozowski, and S. J. Konturek. "Stress and the gut: Pathophysiology, clinical consequences, diagnostic approach and treatment options." *Journal of Physiology and Pharmacology* 62, no. 6 (2011): 591–99.

Krajmalnik-Brown, Rosa, Zehra-Esra Ilhan, Dae-Wook Kang, and John K. DiBaise. "Effects of gut microbes on nutrient absorption and energy regulation." *Nutrition in Clinical Practice* 27, no. 2 (2012): 201–14.

Kuo, Lydia E., Magdalena Czarnecka, Joanna B. Kitlinska, Jason U. Tilan, Richard Kvetňanský, and Zofia Zukowska. "Chronic stress, combined with a high-fat/high-sugar diet, shifts sympathetic signaling toward neuropeptide Y and leads to obesity and the metabolic syndrome." *Annals of the New York Academy of Sciences* 1148, no. 1 (2008): 232–37.

Lally, Phillippa, and Benjamin Gardner. "Promoting habit formation." *Health Psychology Review* 7, suppl. 1 (2013): S137–S158.

Lanou, Amy Joy, Susan E. Berkow, and Neal D. Barnard. "Calcium, dairy products, and bone health in children and young adults: A reevaluation of the evidence." *Pediatrics* 115, no. 3 (2005): 736–43.

Le Chatelier, Emmanuelle, Trine Nielsen, Junjie Qin, Edi Prifti, Falk Hildebrand, Gwen Falony, Mathieu Almeida, et al. "Richness of human gut microbiome correlates with metabolic markers." *Nature* 500, no. 7464 (2013): 541–46.

Lee, Hui Cheng, Andrew M. Jenner, Chin Seng Low, and Yuan Kun Lee. "Effect of tea phenolics and their aromatic fecal bacterial metabolites on intestinal microbiota." *Research in Microbiology* 157, no. 9 (2006): 876–84.

Lenoir, Magalie, Fuschia Serre, Lauriane Cantin, and Serge H. Ahmed. "Intense sweetness surpasses cocaine reward." *PLoS One* 2, no. 8 (2007): e698.

Liju, Vijayasteltar B., Kottarapat Jeena, and Ramadasan Kuttan. "Gastroprotective activity of essential oils from turmeric and ginger." *Journal of Basic and Clinical Physiology and Pharmacology* 26, no. 1 (2015): 95–103.

Lindfors, K., T. Blomqvist, K. Juuti-Uusitalo, S. Stenman, J. Venäläinen, M. Mäki, and K. Kaukinen. "Live probiotic Bifidobacterium lactis bacteria inhibit the toxic effects induced by wheat gliadin in epithelial cell culture." *Clinical & Experimental Immunology* 152, no. 3 (2008): 552–58.

Lopez-Ridaura, Ruy, Walter C. Willett, Eric B. Rimm, Simin Liu, Meir J. Stampfer, JoAnn E. Manson, and Frank B. Hu. "Magnesium intake and risk of type 2 diabetes in men and women." *Diabetes Care* 27, no. 1 (2004): 134–40.

Lyte, Mark. "The microbial organ in the gut as a driver of homeostasis and disease." *Medical Hypotheses* 74, no. 4 (2010): 634–38.

Magis, D. C., B. J. Jandrain, and A. J. Scheen. "Alcohol, insulin sensitivity and diabetes." *Revue Medicale de Liege* 58, no. 7-8 (2002): 501–7.

Manenschijn, Laura, Laura Schaap, N. M. Van Schoor, Suzan van der Pas, G. M. E. E. Peeters, Paul Lips, J. W. Koper, and E. F. C. Van Rossum. "High long-term cortisol levels, measured in scalp hair, are associated with a history of cardiovascular disease." *Journal of Clinical Endocrinology & Metabolism* 98, no. 5 (2013): 2078–83.

Maron, David J. "Flavonoids for reduction of atherosclerotic risk." *Current Atherosclerosis Reports* 6, no. 1 (2004): 73–78.

Marotz, CA, and A. Zarrinpar. "Treating obesity and metabolic syndrome with fecal microbiota transplantation." *Yale Journal of Biology and Medicine* 89(3) (2016), 383–88.

Martinez-Zaguilan, Raul, Elisabeth A. Seftor, Richard EB Seftor, Yi-Wen Chu, Robert J. Gillies, and Mary JC Hendrix. "Acidic pH enhances the invasive behavior of human melanoma cells." *Clinical & Experimental Metastasis* 14, no. 2 (1996): 176–86.

Menke, Andy, Sarah Casagrande, Linda Geiss, and Catherine C. Cowie. "Prevalence of and trends in diabetes among adults in the United States, 1988–2012." *JAMA* 314, no. 10 (2015): 1021–29.

Messaoudi, Michaël, Robert Lalonde, Nicolas Violle, Hervé Javelot, Didier Desor, Amine Nejdi, Jean-François Bisson, et al. "Assessment of psychotropic-like properties of a probiotic formulation (Lactobacillus helveticus R0052 and Bifidobacterium longum R0175) in rats and human subjects." *British Journal of Nutrition* 105, no. 5 (2011): 755–64.

Michaëlsson, Karl, Alicja Wolk, Sophie Langenskiöld, Samar Basu, Eva Warensjö Lemming, Håkan Melhus, and Liisa Byberg. "Milk intake and risk of mortality and fractures in women and men: Cohort studies." *BMJ* 349 (2014): g6015.

"Milk Production 2012." U.S. Department of Agriculture, National Agriculture Statistics Service. July 19, 2012.

Minich, Deanna M., and Jeffrey S. Bland. "Acid-alkaline balance: Role in chronic disease and detoxification." *Alternative Therapies in Health and Medicine* 13, no. 4 (2007): 62.

Mullin, Gerard E. *The Gut Balance Revolution.* New York: Rodale Inc., 2014.

Murray, Michael T., and Joseph E. Pizzorno. *Encyclopedia of Natural Medicine.* 3rd edition. Atria Books, 2012.

Mutlu, Ece A., Patrick M. Gillevet, Huzefa Rangwala, Masoumeh Sikaroodi, Ammar Naqvi, Phillip A. Engen, Mary Kwasny, Cynthia K. Lau, and Ali Keshavarzian.

"Colonic microbiome is altered in alcoholism." *American Journal of Physiology–Gastrointestinal and Liver Physiology* 302, no. 9 (2012): G966–G978.

Naglik, JR, SJ Challacombe, and B Hube. "*Candida albicans* secreted aspartyl proteinases in virulence and pathogenesis." *Microbiology and Molecular Biology Reviews* 67, no. 3 (2003): 400–28. doi:10.1128/MMBR.67.3.400-428.2003. http://www.ncbi.nlm.nih.gov/pmc/articles/PMC193873/.

National Diabetes Statistics Report, 2017. CDC. Accessed March 27, 2018, https://www.cdc.gov/diabetes/pdfs/data/statistics/national-diabetes-statistics-report.pdf.

"Nearly half a million Americans suffered from Clostridium difficile infections in a single year." CDC Newsroom. Accessed March 27, 2018, https://www.cdc.gov/media/releases/2015/p0225-clostridium-difficile.html.

Nesse, Randolph M. "Evolution and addiction." *Addiction* 97, no. 4 (2002): 470–71.

Nestle, Marion. "Diet, Life-style, and Mortality in China: A Study of the Characteristics of 65 Chinese Counties." *BioScience* 41, no. 10 (1991): 725–27.

Nestle, Marion. *Food Politics: How the Food Industry Influences Nutrition and Health.* Vol. 3. Oakland: University of California Press, 2013.

Neuhausen, Susan L., Linda Steele, Sarah Ryan, Maryam Mousavi, Marie Pinto, Kathryn E. Osann, Pamela Flodman, and John J. Zone. "Co-occurrence of celiac disease and other autoimmune diseases in celiacs and their first-degree relatives." *Journal of Autoimmunity* 31, no. 2 (2008): 160–65.

Nidich, Sanford I., Maxwell V. Rainforth, David AF Haaga, John Hagelin, John W. Salerno, Fred Travis, Melissa Tanner, Carolyn Gaylord-King, Sarina Grosswald, and Robert H. Schneider. "A randomized controlled trial on effects of the Transcendental Meditation program on blood pressure, psychological distress, and coping in young adults." *American Journal of Hypertension* 22, no. 12 (2009): 1326–31.

Nielsen, Forrest H. "Ultratrace minerals." *Modern Nutrition in Health and Disease* 8 (1999).

Nilsson, Mikael, Marianne Stenberg, Anders H. Frid, Jens J. Holst, and Inger ME Björck. "Glycemia and insulinemia in healthy subjects after lactose-equivalent meals of milk and other food proteins: The role of plasma amino acids and incretins." *The American Journal of Clinical Nutrition* 80, no. 5 (2004): 1246–53.

Niness, Kathy R. "Inulin and oligofructose: What are they?" *Journal of Nutrition* 129, no. 7 (1999): 1402S–1406S.

Nobile, Clarissa J., and Alexander D. Johnson. "Candida albicans biofilms and human disease." *Annual Review of Microbiology* 69 (2015): 71–92.

Norris, Vic, Franck Molina, and Andrew T. Gewirtz. "Hypothesis: Bacteria control host appetites." *Journal of Bacteriology* 195, no. 3 (2013): 411–16.

Odds, F. C., E. G. Evans, M. A. Taylor, and J. K. Wales. "Prevalence of pathogenic yeasts and humoral antibodies to candida in diabetic patients." *Journal of Clinical Pathology* 31, no. 9 (1978): 840–44.

"The Overuse of Antibiotics in Food Animals Threatens Public Health." Consumers Union: Policy & Action from Consumer Reports. Accessed September 29, 2017, http://consumersunion.org/pdf/Overuse_of_Antibiotics_On_Farms.pdf.

Parlesak, Alexandr, Christian Schäfer, Tatjana Schütz, J. Christian Bode, and Christiane Bode. "Increased intestinal permeability to macromolecules and endotoxemia in patients with chronic alcohol abuse in different stages of alcohol-induced liver disease." *Journal of Hepatology* 32, no. 5 (2000): 742–47.

Préstamo, G., A. Pedrazuela, E. Penas, M. A. Lasunción, and G. Arroyo. "Role of buckwheat diet on rats as prebiotic and healthy food." *Nutrition Research* 23, no. 6 (2003): 803–14.

Qin, Junjie, Ruiqiang Li, Jeroen Raes, Manimozhiyan Arumugam, Kristoffer Solvsten Burgdorf, Chaysavanh Manichanh, Trine Nielsen, et al. "A human gut microbial gene catalogue established by metagenomic sequencing." *Nature* 464, no. 7285 (2010): 59–65.

Rabiu, Bodun A., and Glenn R. Gibson. "Carbohydrates: A limit on bacterial diversity within the colon." *Biological Reviews* 77, no. 3 (2002): 443–53.

Raloff, J. "Hormones: Here's the beef: Environmental concerns reemerge over steroids given to livestock." *Science News* 161, no 1 (2002). Accessed November 21, 2012, https://www.sciencenews.org/article/hormones-heres-beef.

"Recombinant Bovine Growth Hormone." Cancer.org. Accessed July 22, 2015, http://www.cancer.org/cancer/cancercauses/othercarcinogens/athome/recombinant-bovine-growth-hormone.

Remer, Thomas, and Friedrich Manz. "Potential renal acid load of foods and its influence on urine pH." *Journal of the American Dietetic Association* 95, no. 7 (1995): 791–97.

Rizzello, CG, M De Angelis, R Di Cagno, et al. "Highly efficient gluten degradation by lactobacilli and fungal proteases during food processing: New perspectives for celiac disease." *Applied and Environmental Microbiology* 73, no. 14 (2007): 4499–4507. doi:10.1128/AEM.00260-07.

Rolston, KVI, and GP Bodey. "Fungal Infections." In DW Kufe et al., eds. *Holland-Frei Cancer Medicine*, 6th ed. Hamilton, ON: BC Decker, 2003. http://www.ncbi.nlm.nih.gov/books/NBK13518/.

Rubio-Tapia, Alberto, Robert A. Kyle, Edward L. Kaplan, Dwight R. Johnson, William Page, Frederick Erdtmann, Tricia L. Brantner, et al. "Increased prevalence and mortality in undiagnosed celiac disease." *Gastroenterology* 137, no. 1 (2009): 88–93.

Rupp, Rebecca. "Surviving the Sneaky Psychology of Supermarkets." The Plate, *National Geographic*. Accessed December 14, 2017, http://theplate.nationalgeographic.com/2015/06/15/surviving-the-sneaky-psychology-of-supermarkets/.

Saarinen, K., J. Jantunen, and T. Haahtela. "Birch pollen honey for birch pollen allergy—a randomized controlled pilot study." *International Archives of Allergy and Immunology* 155, no. 2 (2011): 160–66.

Samsel, Anthony, and Stephanie Seneff. "Glyphosate's suppression of cytochrome P450 enzymes and amino acid biosynthesis by the gut microbiome: Pathways to modern diseases." *Entropy* 15, no. 4 (2013): 1416–63.

Samsel, Anthony, and Stephanie Seneff. "Glyphosate, pathways to modern diseases II: Celiac sprue and gluten intolerance." *Interdisciplinary Toxicology* 6, no. 4 (2013): 159–84.

Şanlier, Nevin, Büşra Başar Gökcen, and Aybüke Ceyhun Sezgin. "Health benefits of fermented foods." *Critical Reviews in Food Science and Nutrition* (2017): 1–22.

Scarpignato, C. "NSAID-induced intestinal damage: Are luminal bacteria the thera-peutic target?" *Gut* 57, no. 2 (2008): 145–48.

Schley, P. D., and C. J. Field. "The immune-enhancing effects of dietary fibres and prebiotics." *British Journal of Nutrition* 87, no. S2 (2002): S221–S230.

Schmidt, Kristin, Philip J. Cowen, Catherine J. Harmer, George Tzortzis, Steven Errington, and Philip WJ Burnet. "Prebiotic intake reduces the waking cortisol response and alters emotional bias in healthy volunteers." *Psychopharmacology* 232, no. 10 (2015): 1793–1801.

Senapati, T., A. K. Mukerjee, and A. R. Ghosh. "Observations on the effect of glyphosate based herbicide on ultra structure (SEM) and enzymatic activity in dif-ferent regions of alimentary canal and gill of Channa punctatus (Bloch)." *Journal of Crop and Weed* 5, no. 1 (2009): 236–45.

Sender, Ron, Shai Fuchs, and Ron Milo. "Revised estimates for the number of human and bacteria cells in the body." *PLoS Biology* 14, no. 8 (2016): e1002533.

Singleton, Omar, Britta K. Hölzel, Mark Vangel, Narayan Brach, James Carmody, and Sara W. Lazar. "Change in brainstem gray matter concentration following a mindfulness-based intervention is correlated with improvement in psychological well-being." *Frontiers in Human Neuroscience* 8 (2014).

Smith, Bob L. "Organic foods vs. supermarket foods: Element levels." *Journal of Ap-plied Nutrition* 45, no. 1 (1993): 35–39.

Sonnenburg, Justin, and Erica Sonnenburg. *The Good Gut: Taking Control of Your Weight, Your Mood, and Your Long Term Health.* Penguin, 2015, 71.

Spreadbury, Ian. "Comparison with ancestral diets suggests dense acellular carbohy-drates promote an inflammatory microbiota, and may be the primary dietary cause of leptin resistance and obesity." *Diabetes, Metabolic Syndrome and Obesity: Targets and Therapy* 5 (2012): 175.

Swithers, Susan E. "Artificial sweeteners produce the counterintuitive effect of induc-ing metabolic derangements." *Trends in Endocrinology & Metabolism* 24, no. 9 (2013): 431–41.

Swithers, Susan E., and Terry L. Davidson. "A role for sweet taste: Calorie predictive relations in energy regulation by rats." *Behavioral Neuroscience* 122, no. 1 (2008): 161.

Tang, Yi-Yuan, Yinghua Ma, Yaxin Fan, Hongbo Feng, Junhong Wang, Shigang Feng, Qilin Lu, et al. "Central and autonomic nervous system interaction is altered by short-term meditation." *Proceedings of the National Academy of Sciences* 106, no. 22 (2009): 8865–70.

Tietjen, G. E., M. Karmakar, and A. A. Amialchuk. "CRP and migraine in young adults: Results from the ADD health study." In *Headache*, vol. 56, no. 8 (2016): 1397.

Townshend, Julia, and Theodora Duka. "Attentional bias associated with alcohol cues: Differences between heavy and occasional social drinkers." *Psychopharmacology* 157, no. 1 (2001): 67–74.

Tryon, Matthew S., Kimber L. Stanhope, Elissa S. Epel, Ashley E. Mason, Rashida Brown, Valentina Medici, Peter J. Havel, and Kevin D. Laugero. "Excessive sugar consumption may be a difficult habit to break: A view from the brain and body." *Journal of Clinical Endocrinology & Metabolism* 100, no. 6 (2015): 2239–47.

Tuohy, Kieran M., Lorenza Conterno, Mattia Gasperotti, and Roberto Viola. "Up-regulating the human intestinal microbiome using whole plant foods, polyphenols, and/or fiber." *Journal of Agricultural and Food Chemistry* 60, no. 36 (2012): 8776–82.

Turner, Andrew G., Paul H. Anderson, and Howard A. Morris. "Vitamin D and bone health." *Scandinavian Journal of Clinical and Laboratory Investigation* 72, suppl. 243 (2012): 65–72.

Turta, Olli, and Samuli Rautava. "Antibiotics, obesity and the link to microbes—what are we doing to our children?" *BMC Medicine* 14, no. 1 (2016): 57.

Ukiya, Motohiko, Toshihiro Akihisa, Harukuni Tokuda, Masakazu Toriumi, Teruo Mukainaka, Norihiro Banno, Yumiko Kimura, Jun-ichi Hasegawa, and Hoyoku Nishino. "Inhibitory effects of cucurbitane glycosides and other triterpenoids from the fruit of *Momordica grosvenori* on Epstein-Barr virus early antigen induced by tumor promoter 12-O-tetradecanoylphorbol-13-acetate." *Journal of Agricultural and Food Chemistry* 50, no. 23 (2002): 6710–15.

Urita, Yoshihisa, Motonobu Sugimoto, Kazuo Hike, Naotaka Torii, Yoshinori Kikuchi, Hidenori Kurakata, Eiko Kanda, Masahiko Sasajima, and Kazumasa Miki. "High incidence of fermentation in the digestive tract in patients with reflux oesophagitis." *European Journal of Gastroenterology & Hepatology* 18, no. 5 (2006): 531–35.

Vane, John, and Regina Botting. "Inflammation and the mechanism of action of anti-inflammatory drugs." *FASEB Journal* 1, no. 2 (1987): 89–96.

Vázquez-González, Denisse, Ana María Perusquía-Ortiz, Max Hundeiker, and Alexandro Bonifaz. "Opportunistic yeast infections: Candidiasis, cryptococcosis, trichosporonosis and geotrichosis." *Journal der Deutschen Dermatologischen Gesellschaft* 11, no. 5 (2013): 381–94.

"Vitamin B12 Deficiency Anemia." Johns Hopkins Medical Health Library. Accessed September 1, 2017, http://www.hopkinsmedicine.org/healthlibrary/conditions/hematology_and_blood_disorders/anemia_of_b12_deficiency_pernicious_anemia_85,P00080/.

Webb, Bradley A., Michael Chimenti, Matthew P. Jacobson, and Diane L. Barber. "Dysregulated pH: A perfect storm for cancer progression." *Nature Reviews Cancer* 11, no. 9 (2011): 671.

Wetherell, Julie Loebach, Lin Liu, Thomas L. Patterson, Niloofar Afari, Catherine R. Ayers, Steven R. Thorp, Jill A. Stoddard, et al. "Acceptance and commitment therapy for generalized anxiety disorder in older adults: A preliminary report." *Behavior Therapy* 42, no. 1 (2011): 127–34.

Wetherell, Julie Loebach, Niloofar Afari, Thomas Rutledge, John T. Sorrell, Jill A. Stoddard, Andrew J. Petkus, Brittany C. Solomon, et al. "A randomized, controlled trial of acceptance and commitment therapy and cognitive-behavioral therapy for chronic pain." *Pain* 152, no. 9 (2011): 2098–2107.

"What the World Eats." *National Geographic*. Accessed December 14, 2017, https://www.nationalgeographic.com/what-the-world-eats/.

Whorwell, Peter J., Linda Altringer, Jorge Morel, Yvonne Bond, Duane Charbonneau, Liam O'Mahony, Barry Kiely, Fergus Shanahan, and Eamonn MM Quigley. "Efficacy of an encapsulated probiotic Bifidobacterium infantis 35624 in women with irritable bowel syndrome." *American Journal of Gastroenterology* 101, no. 7 (2006): 1581–90.

Williams, Gary M., Robert Kroes, and Ian C. Munro. "Safety evaluation and risk assessment of the herbicide Roundup and its active ingredient, glyphosate, for humans." *Regulatory Toxicology and Pharmacology* 31, no. 2 (2000): 117–65.

Wong, Julia MW, Russell De Souza, Cyril WC Kendall, Azadeh Emam, and David JA Jenkins. "Colonic health: Fermentation and short chain fatty acids." *Journal of Clinical Gastroenterology* 40, no. 3 (2006): 235–43.

Xu, Q., S. Y. Chen, L. D. Deng, L. P. Feng, L. Z. Huang, and R. R. Yu. "Antioxidant effect of mogrosides against oxidative stress induced by palmitic acid in mouse insulinoma NIT-1 cells." *Brazilian Journal of Medical and Biological Research* 46, no. 11 (2013): 949–55.

Yemma, J. J., and M. P. Berk. "Chemical and physiological effects of Candida albicans toxin on tissues." *Cytobios* 77, no. 310 (1993): 147–158.

Zhou, Albert Lihong, Nancie Hergert, Giovanni Rompato, and Michael Lefevre. "Whole grain oats improve insulin sensitivity and plasma cholesterol profile and modify gut microbiota composition in C57BL/6J mice–3." *Journal of Nutrition* 145, no. 2 (2014): 222–30.

Index

About the Author

Heather A. Wise, M.P.H., is a wellness consultant, health coach, and avid food fermenter. She started her own wellness coaching business, The Smart Palate, and has given a number of workshops and talks on gut health and wellness, including at Harvard Medical School. Heather lives with her family in the Boston area.